Other books by Philip Burnard

- Experimental Learning in Action
- Perceptions of AIDS Counselling: a View from Health Professionals and AIDS Counsellors
- Self Disclosure: A Contemporary Analysis (with P. Morrison)
- Women and AIDS in Rural Africa (with G. Mwale)
- Aspects of Forensic Psychiatric Nursing (with P. Morrison)
- Spirituality and Nursing Practice (with J. Harrison)
- Professional and Ethical Issues in Nursing: The Code of Professional Conduct (with C. M. Chapman)
- Counselling Skills for Health Professionals
- Teaching Interpersonal Skills: A Handbook of Experiential Learning for Health Professionals
- Nurse Education: The Way Forward (with C. M. Chapman)
- Nursing Research in Action: Developing Basic Skills (with P. Morrison)
- Coping with Stress in the Health Professions: a Practical Guide
- Caring and Communicating: The Interpersonal Relationship in Nursing (with P. Morrison)
- Caring and Communicating: Facilitators' Manual (with P. Morrison)
- Effective Communication Skills for Health Professionals
- Know Yourself! Self-Awareness Activities for Nurses
- Communicate! Communication Skills for Health Workers
- Interpersonal Skills Training: A Sourcebook of Activities for Trainers
- Counselling: A Guide to Practice in Nursing
- Writing for Health Professionals: A Manual for Writers
- Counselling Skills: A Sourcebook of Activities for Trainers
- What is Counselling?
- Personal Computing for Health Professionals
- Health Care Computing: A Survival Guide for PC Users
- Survival Guide for Nursing Students
- Critical Care Nursing (with B. Millar)

NURSES COUNSELLING

The View from the Practitioners

Edited by

PHILIP BURNARD

PhD, MSc, RMN, RGN, DipN, CertEd, RNT

Programme Manager
BSc (Hons) Nursing Studies
University of Wales College of Medicine
Cardiff

and

IAN HULATT

MSc, RGN, RMN, DipN, CertEd(FE), DipCouns, RNT

Lecturer, Advanced Nursing Section
South East Wales Institute of Nursing and Midwifery Education
Cardiff

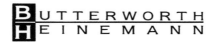

BUTTERWORTH
HEINEMANN

Butterworth-Heinemann
Linacre House, Jordan Hill, Oxford OX2 8DP
A division of Reed Educational and Professional Publishing Ltd

ℛ A member of the Reed Elsevier plc group

OXFORD   BOSTON   JOHANNESBURG
MELBOURNE   NEW DELHI   SINGAPORE

First published 1996

© Reed Educational and Professional Publishing Ltd 1996

British Library Cataloguing in Publication Data
Nurses counselling: the view from the practitioners
    1 Counselors   2 Patients – Counselling of   3 Nurse and patient
    I Burnard, Philip   II Hulatt, Ian
    362.1'04256

ISBN 0 7506 2004 8

Library of Congress Cataloguing in Publication Data
Nurses counselling: the view from the practitioners/edited by
    Philip Burnard and Ian Hulatt.
    p.   cm.
    Includes bibliographical references and index.
    ISBN 0 7506 2004 8
    1 Nursing – Psychological aspects.   2 Counseling.   3 Nurse and
    patient.   I Burnard, Philip.   II Hulatt, Ian.
    [DNLM: 1 Nursing.   2 Counseling. WY 87 N97445]
    RT86.N875
    610.73–dc20   96–14626
                                                          CIP

Typesetting by David Gregson Associates, Beccles, Suffolk
Printed and bound in Great Britain by
Biddles Ltd, Guildford and King's Lynn

CONTENTS

LIST OF CONTRIBUTORS

Peter Akinwunmi MBA, BSc(Hons), PGCertEd, RMN, RNT
Peter Akinwunmi is Curriculum Development Manager, South East Wales Institute of Nursing and Midwifery Education, University of Wales College of Medicine. He has been lecturing on transcultural counselling and related issues since 1988. He is a member of anti-racist and multicultural interest groups. His experience as a sports psychologist since 1990 has furthered his knowledge and interest in transcultural counselling. His current study of clinical theology is leading him to examine the influence of spirituality and faith on athletic performance.

Philip J. Barker PhD, RN
Phil Barker is Professor of Psychiatric Nursing Practice at the University of Newcastle-upon-Tyne. Previously he was Director of Studies at the Department of Psychiatry, University of Dundee. He has been involved in counselling and psychotherapy since the mid-1970s, across a wide range of clinical settings – from the experience of addiction to the experience of psychosis.

Philip Burnard PhD, MSc, RGN, RMN, DipN, CertEd, RNT
Philip Burnard is Reader in the School of Nursing Studies at the University of Wales College of Medicine. He has run counselling workshops in a variety of European and Far Eastern countries, is the author of many books on counselling and communication and has undertaken research into nurses' attitudes towards client-centred counselling, communication and counselling skills.

Mary Chambers DPhil, BEd, RGN, RMN, RCNT, RNT, DN(Lond), CertBehPsychotherapy
Mary Chambers is Senior Lecturer with special responsibility

for developing clinically-based mental health nursing courses, for example, Cognitive Behavioural Psychotherapy at the University of Ulster at Coleraine, Northern Ireland. Her research interests include the educational preparation of mental health nurses and the effectiveness of psychiatric nursing interventions.

Ian Hulatt MSc, RGN, RMN, DipN, CertEd (FE), RNT, DipCouns

Ian Hulatt is Programme Manager of the BSc Nursing Studies programme in the South East Wales Institute of Nursing and Midwifery, University of Wales College of Medicine. A practising counsellor and registered teacher with the Central School for Counselling Therapy, he has taught counselling theory and skills to a variety of professional groups.

Alun Jones MA, RMN, RGN, CPN Cert, DIPN (Pt a), DipPsych (UKCP), PGDE, RNT

Alun Jones is a lecturer at the School of Nursing Studies, University of Manchester. Alun is a psychodynamic counsellor, UKCP registered. His experience as a counsellor includes working in a general hospital and community medical settings. Alun has experience of teaching counselling modules related to a wide range of nursing specialties and has been a member of both the 'Training' and 'Hospital setting' sub committies of the British Association for Counselling. He is currently engaged in research and regularly facilitates workshops related to counselling and psychotherapy.

Jim Richardson BA, RGN, RSCN, PCGE

Jim Richardson is a lecturer in nursing at the School of Nursing Studies, University of Wales College of Medicine, Cardiff. He trained as a general and paediatric nurse in Aberdeen and London. He practised as a nurse in child health settings in Finland and Wales. He is currently engaged in child health nurse education and his interests include cultural issues in child health care and the effects of chronic childhood illness on the family.

Colin D. Somerville RGN, RMN, DipCllgSkills (SWLC), DipAdlerianCllg (11P), Adlerian Accredited Counsellor (ASIP), BAC Accredited Counsellor (1984–94)

Colin Somerville was born in England but raised and educated in New Zealand. In 1962 he returned to England to test his vocation to the religious life during which time he trained as a general nurse. He left the religious life in 1976 and trained as a psychiatric nurse. He began counselling training in 1980 and now holds two counselling diplomas. From 1982–1993 he was a counsellor for nurses with the Royal College of Nursing. He was an accredited counsellor with the British Association for Counselling from 1984–1994 and is a member of the Council of the Adlerian Society of Great Britain. He works for the Lesbian and Gay Christian movement and, on a voluntary basis, for the Sussex Beacon, which is a continuing care centre for people living with HIV and AIDS.

Marie Toman MN, RMN, CertEd, RNT

Marie Toman is a lecturer practitioner in Forensic Psychiatry at the Caswell Clinic, Bridgend, Mid Glamorgan. Her experience is rooted in acute psychiatry and she became a nurse lecturer in 1986. Her research interests are in the forensic psychiatric nurse's role, with special interest in assessing risk and dangerousness, and with the many, complex issues forensic nurses encounter when counselling mentally disordered offenders.

Allison J. Williams BSc, RGN, PGCE

Allison Williams undertook a combined BSc/RGN course at South Bank Polytechnic. She worked at Southampton University as a lecturer in nursing and is now employed as a Clinical Nurse Specialist in Genetics at the Wales Genetics Services, University of Wales Hospital Trust, Cardiff.

Bob Wright Hon MSc, RGN, RMN

Bob Wright is Clinical Nurse Specialist in Crisis Care in the Accident and Emergency Department at Leeds General Infirmary. He previously worked as a Charge Nurse in Accident and Emergency and in Psychiatry. Part of his role involves debriefing critical incidents and disasterous events.

INTRODUCTION

Counselling has become part of what nurses do. That is not to say that the term 'counselling' or the process of counselling are not problematic. Over the past few years, many have questioned the validity and appropriateness of counselling, both within and outside of nursing. There are also very few books about *how counselling is done*. While there are many texts on the theory and practice of counselling, not many offer glimpses of what goes on when people do counselling.

In this book, we have tried to offer a range of views of what nurse-counsellors do and how they describe what they do. We invited a range of practitioners to contribute chapters on a variety of different themes. We asked them to write about their own approaches to both the theory and practice of counselling and invited them to give examples of how all this works in practice.

In the opening chapter, we offer a discussion about the range and breadth of counselling as it relates to nursing. This is a critical discussion and seeks to highlight some of the problems of counselling and of doing research in this field.

In Chapter 2, Philip Barker – an experienced and skilled teacher and therapist – describes his own approach to doing counselling with the aim of affecting behavioural change. He has often sought to integrate various approaches and theories into his work and this is reflected in the chapter.

In Chapter 3, Allison Williams offers a view of counselling from the point of view of genetics. This is an area that is usually thought of as 'medical' and it is interesting to see the field from a *nursing* point of view.

In Chapter 4, Jim Richardson offers a discussion about talking with children and suggests that he prefers the idea of 'talking with' to 'counselling'. He illustrates some of the pitfalls and problems of adults communicating with children and offers concrete advice.

In Chapter 5, the nurse – him or herself – comes into the picture and Colin Somerville describes his own particular approach to counselling nurses, using an Adlerian approach.

In Chapter 6, Mary Chambers – who has conducted research in the field of nurse education and communication – offers her own view of counselling in mental health settings.

In Chapter 7, Marie Toman discusses her approach to counselling in the forensic nursing arena. This is a specialized field, within the larger field of psychiatric nursing and one that has only recently gained recognition as an emerging speciality.

In Chapter 8, Bob Wright, an internationally recognized nurse counsellor offers a detailed description and discussion about counselling those in crisis and describes, too, the practical skills involved in counselling those who suffer post-traumatic stress.

In Chapter 9, Alun Jones offers a valuable discussion of approaches to bereavement counselling (Taking Counsel: *Nursing Times*, **90**, No 26, 28–29). The final chapter, by Peter Akinwunmi, offers a review of some of the issues of counselling and racism. In today's multicultural society, nurses would do well to review their own views on this issue.

Counselling is all about communicating with other people. In this book, we have encouraged the chapter authors to offer their own views, in their own ways. We do not believe that there is one *right* way to counsel and we hope that the contributions in this book offer something of the richness that various people bring both to the nursing profession and to the practice of counselling.

1

Counselling in Nursing

Philip Burnard and Ian Hulatt

Nursing is an interpersonal profession. It involves people caring for other people and part of that caring includes talking about problems and difficulties. Sometimes, this talking process amounts to counselling. What makes the field difficult is that there is not a general consensus about what *constitutes* counselling. There are not only theoretical differences, there are also differences of opinion about how and when counselling should be carried out and by whom it should be practised.

In recent years, there has been considerable controversy about whether or not counselling 'works'. Some claim that counselling is no more effective than no treatment or therapy at all. At the other end of the spectrum, many 'alternative' or 'complementary' therapists would claim that no 'proof' of efficacy is necessary: what counts is that people *say* that it helps. This, arguably, is the pragmatic view: that any activity that people find useful is a valuable activity in and of itself, as long as it is not actively harming those people. In this chapter, we explore some of the features that go to make up what many people would feel to be the essential elements of counselling. As we have suggested, this is no easy task. As this book will reveal, there are many approaches, many theories and many ways of practising. We also feel that this is a good thing. In the absence of concrete evidence of what does and does not make a measurable difference to patients, it seems good that there is a range of possibilities from which those patients may choose. And *choice*, perhaps, should be the issue. It seems both morally inappropriate and practically inadvisable to attempt to force any one approach on other people. In a health service which aims at choice and independence, it is surely important that people – both patients and staff – are able to choose with some awareness, the sort of counselling approach that they feel would most likely suit their temperament, belief system and general approach to life. We acknowledge that this is unlikely always to be possible but it does seem to point to the notion of 'transparency' in counselling practice. Counsellors should, perhaps, make it clear to their clients what they can expect from counselling, both in terms of the counsellor's general approach and – possibly – in terms of outcomes (although this later point is a particularly difficult one and one that makes 'outcome research' so difficult).

Counselling is a reasonably recent phenomenon. It might be claimed that it was 'invented' by Carl Rogers, American psychotherapist and progressive educator (Rogers, 1951, 1983). In the late 1940s, Rogers was practising what he called *educational therapy*. He felt that the best way to help parents who had difficulties with their children was to supply those parents with the most up-to-date psychological information available, so that they could make informed decisions about how to help their own children. What Rogers found, however, was that parents sometimes did and sometimes did not *use* that information. As a result of considerable thought about the matter, Rogers chose to switch the focus of his work *away* from information-giving and towards helping people to make their *own* decisions. This was due, in part, to Rogers losing his religious convictions and moving towards a greater belief in an 'existential' view of life (Kirschenbaum, 1978).

Out of all this was born what came to be known, at first, as non-directive counselling and later as *client-centred* therapy. Rogers' counselling style depended, heavily, on avoiding information giving, allowing people to identify and clarify their own problems and in enabling them to find their own solutions to those problems.

Rogers' approach was pervasive and over the next few decades, the client-centred approach, arguably become the most common approach to 'doing' counselling. It affected the whole range of counselling activities from marriage guidance to educational counselling. The client-centred approach was reasonably easy to teach and fairly easy to learn. It did not depend on a particularly complicated theory base and it was optimistic in its foundation in Rogers' belief that people, given the chance, would change their behaviour towards that which was positive and life-enhancing. In this sense, the approach was very 'American': it emphasized the positive, down-played the negative and encouraged a belief in the individual's ability to sort themselves out. It also removed, at a stroke, the need for a professional 'expert'. Experts, such as they were, were fairly easily trained and could practise the client-centred approach to counselling alongside a range of other health care activities.

The client-centred approach to counselling could then be found in a range of texts related to interpersonal skills in nursing. The approach became a popular one with nurses and with nurse educators and this remains the case today. The argument is often that the client-centred approach belongs to another generation: a generation in which there was prosperity, financial security and a more liberal set of values in operation. The client-centred approach with its belief in the client as a potentially fully functioning person (Rogers, 1961; Mearns and Thorne, 1988) and a dogged determination of the therapist to remain non-directive has not remained unchallenged.

Further developments in 1960s' America included the practice of Gestalt therapy with its focus on creating a true encounter between therapist and client. The peeling away of any phoniness (Perls, 1969) in the client was achieved by the use of techniques such as the hot seat. Such confrontational methods and the pursuit of polarities in the client are clear evidence of a shift from the warmth and empathy synonymous with the client-centred approach. Once again a way of working with individuals or groups had become synonymous with an individual. This time it was the charismatic Fritz Perl with his kaftan robes, long hair and flowing white beard.

Other approaches have focused on different aspects of psychological life. Berne (1964) examined the interactive nature of humans and how they encounter each other following internal scripts. The notion of games and the patterns of interaction became the focus of therapy, with the helper bringing the client to an awareness of their manifestation in everyday life.

The move in emphasis from the client's feelings to his/her thoughts has found expression in the work of Cognitive therapists such as Beck (1976). This more analytical way of working has proven popular with those who attempt to help individuals who are labelled depressed. Based upon the notion that one's internal talk can affect mood, the therapist works with the messages that the client gives to him/herself. These ways of thinking may have their own origins in early development (being told you are stupid rather than doing something stupid). Subsequent normal disappointments in life may be interpreted within the context of the negative belief. Thus the negative belief is seen to be reinforced (or proven). By learning new patterns of thinking, the client learns to challenge internal negative talk. This may be achieved by simple requests to the client to provide evidence for a belief, therefore exposing its irrationality. An example would be a client who states they are always kept waiting in shops. However, on exploration the therapist determines the shop was busy for everybody. This approach has been further refined with the addition of a behavioural component. The cognitive-behavioural style of working (Trower *et al.*, 1988) has seen the addition of the notion of homework for the client. Believing that action is a central component (and one omitted from the client-centred approach), clients are given homework that then affords them the opportunity to try out new strategies for living.

If the spirit of the age can be considered to have had an influence upon client-centred therapy then this process certainly continues today. Health care is becoming increasingly focused on the measurable outcome of any intervention. This process is being applied to the phenomenon of counselling. However, outcomes are notoriously difficult to measure in this arena. Within primary care settings a broadly utilitarian approach to the rationing of therapy is occurring. This would seem to be based on the belief that if client change can occur after six sessions, then why not give only six sessions to more clients. Of course this could be contrary to current trends in consumer choice.

Approaches such as brief therapy (De Shazer, 1985) can be used in this context. This is again a way of working with clients that focuses on outcomes, to the almost total exclusion of consideration of the therapeutic relationship.

If theoretical perspectives can be seen as constantly evolving, some issues have a certain permanence. One such issue would be whether there is any difference between counselling and psychotherapy. We would consider that there are probably more similarities than differences, and that the differences are more than just the financial cost!

Similarities would certainly include the importance of entering the client's frame of reference. Also the centrality of the therapeutic relationship is common to most schools of helping. This is true whether the 'here and now' of the relationship is said to mirror the 'there and then', or is the vehicle to convey the therapeutic use of self. Other areas of agreement would possibly include the special nature of the time together, and the boundaries that surround it. These would include confidentiality and the levels of disclosure on the part of the therapist.

Differences do exist in areas of emphasis however. Training in psychotherapy tends to be longer, and grounded in one approach. There is also an increased expectancy that the trainee will be in therapy himself, which will underpin his practice and education. The depth of the work with the client tends to be deeper, moving from presenting issues to aspects of self at a more profound level.

We would suggest that counselling and psychotherapy are on a continuum, and that practitioners move along this continuum at times. Where the two ways of working are identical is in the recognition of the essential nature of supervision (Houston, 1990; Holloway, 1994). This process (currently being adopted into mainstream nursing circles) provides not only education for the therapist, but protection for the client.

Supervision is all the more important because counselling and psychotherapy are both unregulated. The absence of any regulatory body has resulted in a proliferation of training courses and practitioners. Therefore it is essential that counsellors or psychotherapists seek formal opportunities to discuss and review their work. Responsible practitioners are expected to undergo supervision; indeed some agencies make this a formal requirement of their workers.

Counselling can therefore be described as an activity which possesses central values and characteristics of practice, which are expressed within a variety of theoretical frameworks. For clients this affords the opportunity to find the approach which they are most comfortable with. Counselling is of a very personal nature, therefore it is important that clients are not only comfortable with their therapist, but also the way they will be working together.

In the chapters that follow the authors will be describing how they work with clients. They will be describing what they believe to be the 'best fit in their respective fields of practice'.

2

Counselling for Behavioural Change

Philip J. Barker

Introduction

It has become increasingly popular to assert that all forms of counselling and psychotherapy involve a covert manipulation of disadvantaged people (Masson, 1989). In a similar vein it has been suggested that the assumption that any form of counselling or therapy can be of 'use' is inherently flawed (Smail, 1987). Despite some sympathy for the rationales supporting these views, I believe that the analysis may be correct but the conclusions ill-founded. Any form of counselling or psychotherapy may be used against the best interests of the person. Equally, many therapists may be unable to offer any significant form of help to distressed people: whether this is a function of the methods used or of non-specific therapist characteristics is difficult to say. I operate from the assumption, however, that people who experience mental distress, of any kind, may be helped to reduce this experience of distress. The extent to which this is possible, how it might be accomplished and by whom, can only be concluded in retrospect: after the event. This chapter summarizes some of the assumptions which I have developed about counselling which are based on such post hoc analyses. My assumptions about the nature of counselling are not, however, cast in any concrete mode, and need to be modified, constantly, in the light of the experience gained from the counselling relationship. Counselling is a process which goes on between people. It is not something which is done to people called patients. It is assumed that counselling is about helping people to address problems in their lives and to begin (at least) the independent process of living life more constructively. Despite the dangers of 'political incorrectness' I shall assume that those who are counselled are 'suffering' some form of distress and, as such, will be referred to throughout as patients using the female gender for convenience; the male gender being retained for the description of counsellor.

Counselling is a two-way educational process. The people defined as counsellor and patient learn, through collaboration, more about the problem, its nature, and how it might be addressed. Where counselling fails to achieve its goals one must assume that one or both of the parties is not making full use of the 'mutual learning' process. I consider it necessary to note that, in many instances, the failure to exploit 'mutual learning' is more important to the success of counselling, than the theory underpinning the counselling method.

Counselling for behaviour change

The counselling approach addressed within this chapter might be classed as spiritual in character: it deals with what people might become, rather than with any notion of who people are, or where people might have come from – the latter might be characterized as an enduring feature of forms of counselling deriving from psychoanalytic theories. The approach discussed here emphasizes the choosing potential of individuals: the main thrust of counselling is to draw attention to the core function of choice, on a day-to-day, moment-by-moment basis, and to extend the person's exercise of control over the choices she makes. It is not assumed that the simple exercise of choice will revolutionize a person's life. Rather, it is assumed that the recognition of her choosing nature will represent a first step toward a fuller, more effective, less dysfunctional, life ahead. Counselling aims to help the person recognize what may be changed and how; and what must be left for acceptance.

The major assumption within this approach is that any significant – i.e. meaningful for the person – change can arise only from the complex interaction of action and reflection. Sometimes the action is planned; at other times arbitrary. Similarly reflection can follow or preface action. In all cases, however, they are inextricably linked: the ubiquitous double act of human development.

The counselling approach addressed in this chapter is described primarily in terms of the nature of the helping relationship: counselling is assumed to be mainly about helping someone to review a specific life situation, consider, and (perhaps) to enact options. The counsellor is under no obligation to 'change' the person. It is assumed that the person is in a constant process of change anyway. Counselling serves as a setting within which the person can develop awareness of this process and has an opportunity to extend further the sense of being able to select and determine, to some extent, the direction of such changes. Much of Western psychology has operated on the notion that the 'real person' lies in the subconscious, masked by a false self which can crack under stress, allowing the real self to show itself. The complexities of the 'false–real self' debate will not be addressed here. It will be assumed instead that all people possess 'multiple selves', each of which is real in the context within which it is present. The person who presents within counselling as 'a hopeless case', or who is 'unlovable' is describing different notions of self. Given that others may have found it difficult to recognize these two particular 'selves', the counsellor's aim is to facilitate the person's recognition of which other selves might be being perceived by others. This approach encourages the view that people are multidimensional, rather than any single 'personality' or 'type'. Recognition of these varieties, or dimensions (the distinction is unimportant), of the 'self' may provide the person with a sense of freedom previously not apparent.

In this sense the counsellor will focus attention upon how the person shifts, perhaps imperceptibly, from one 'self' to another: these shifts are most apparent through changes in behaviour. The counsellor does not believe that behaviour is all. Rather, the counsellor will explore with the person the view that her behaviour is all that makes a mark in the world. For instance, is it sufficient to 'think kind thoughts' or to 'feel kindness towards others'? How do such thoughts and feelings stand compared to acts of kindness? The counsellor operates from the assumption (which cannot be verified or contradicted) that people grow through their behaviour; and that such acts, reflexively, shape feelings and thoughts.

Counsel for whom?

The counselling approach described here is appropriate for a wide range of people. Indeed, it is easier to suggest for whom it might not be appropriate: those who seek to understand the origins of their mental distress, especially through exploration of their early experiences. This approach may also be unpalatable for people who choose to believe that their problems are primarily a function of external sources. Paradoxically, such people can often benefit from the 'empowering' nature of this approach. This form of counselling is appropriate for people who wish to reinforce the possession of their own lives; who recognize, to some extent, that they are responsible individuals and, as such, need to take direct action to resolve the problems which confront them in their lives. People who are experiencing relationship problems, with others or with themselves, are primary candidates. People who have been injured through their experience of others, especially through abusive relationships, and who have developed self-defeating views of themselves or others in their world, are also appropriate subjects. Some of these people might be described as 'the worried well' or 'the psychotically disturbed'. Once the counsellor moves from classification to a consideration of human themes these distinctions lose their potency.

The approach is largely disinterested in describing people in traditional diagnostic terms: depressed, anxious, bereaved, etc. Instead, the focus is upon how people act: people who say that they believe (for instance) that they are no good, incompetent, have no future or will never do this or that; people who say that they feel powerless, fearful, victimized, put upon, etc. The emphasis upon what people say is central: the counsellor has no way of knowing the person's internal experience, but takes what she says on trust. By so doing he offers her an opportunity to begin to examine how she has constructed the experience of powerlessness (for example): what does it mean to her; how does she know that she is powerless; when is she **not** powerless?

Background

I assume that the helping relationship, which is the very core of counselling, involves the judicious use of the following four principles. These are expressed in terms of the needs for:

1. A well-planned rationale: the counsellor needs to offer the person an appropriate perspective on the counselling process, how this will relate to her life problems under review, and how this will affect the emergent counsellor–patient relationship. This rationale threads its way throughout the whole counselling relationship.
2. Thinking skills training: the counsellor needs to help the person 'sharpen' her awareness of the construction of 'problems' and, by consequence, her potential (in cognitive terms) to deconstruct, reconstruct or otherwise resolve those problems through the discovery of solutions.
3. Generalization: the counselling context is used as a preparation, or coaching scenario. Counselling has no point in itself: it is merely a way-station – a stage on the person's exploration of alternative ways of living in life.
4. Re-shaping beliefs: the person who enters counselling brings a certain set of beliefs about herself, her world and her options for change. The process of counselling involves addressing some of these beliefs with a view to helping her reshape these 'self-constructions': developing schemas which are potentially more flexible, adaptive, self-supportive and which, most importantly, might serve as a basis for negotiating behavioural change.

Emphasis upon action

The counselling approach described here centres upon the assumption that change is achieved through action (or behaviour). I agree with Reynolds' view that people with psychological problems (which means all of us at some time or another) 'feel and think a great deal and do very little' (Reynolds and Cormack, 1985). As a result, the interaction between counsellor and patient serves only as a part of the planning or rehearsal for the enaction of behaviour change. The many influences of philosophy and technique represent only some of the possible, theoretically infinite, means towards the end of behaviour change.

The counselling base

What is counselling for? What are its aims? What does the coun-sellor expect will happen? How might these expectations be shared with the person being counselled? It is assumed that counselling is an extraordinary interpersonal situation where two or more people, working intimately or in a group, examine some life experiences, deemed to be important by the person being counselled. It is assumed that the person entering the counselling relationship knows the nature of these problems. The counselling process is largely concerned with exploring her current understanding of these problems, with a view to beginning to change them. The counselling process is relatively open-ended but is based upon a recognizable structure.

Exploring expectations

The person needs to be introduced to the counselling process. This should begin with an initiation to discuss her thoughts and feelings about entering this extraordinary relationship. What does she think the counsellor might be able to do for her? How does she feel about exposing herself, aspects of her life, to a rel-ative stranger? Some time needs to be set aside at the outset for clarification of these thoughts and feelings. If she has un-realistic expectations, it is necessary to clarify what is, or is not, on offer. The counsellor may suggest that some of the concerns about self-exploration, self-examination, self-management (etc.) might be carried forward to form part of the counselling agenda. It may suffice, however, simply to acknowledge that the person is entering a relationship which might pose a significant emotional 'threat'.

Counsellor: (continuing) How do you feel about discussing your problems with me ... with a man?
Patient: Oh I don't know. Its very difficult ... embarrassing ... Well I suppose I knew it would be tough.
Counsellor: What: You knew I would be tough?
Patient: No! (laughs) I mean, ... Oh, I guess, I knew I would find it hard to get down to dealing with all of this stuff.
Counsellor: No pain no gain?
Patient: Perhaps.

Counsellor: Fine. Maybe we only know what things are like when we look back. I hope you will tell me how it feels as we go along. I expect you to keep me on track. You have lived with yourself all your life. You will help me greatly if you keep reminding yourself that I am trying to work out who you are. If it's any consolation I'm not sure what will happen here either, but I'm looking forward to finding out. Let's talk about where we might begin.

Negotiating the relationship

Some discussion of the practical arrangements is also necessary. The timetabling for the sessions (how often, where, when and for how long) provides a useful starting point for negotiating the relationship. This allows the person to express preferences, while allowing the counsellor to state the 'possibilities'. This adds to the scene setting, taking it a stage further into the realms of adult, egalitarian negotiation. The aim is to give the person the clear impression that, from the outset, she will be consulted, but that it may not be possible to meet her every wish. Hopefully she will gain an impression of an equal, dignified relationship.

The person might be forgiven for thinking that much of this negotiation is no more than politeness. It may be appropriate, therefore, to offer the person some specific power, to use within the session. Giving her control over the time available may be an appropriate strategy[1].

Counsellor: (after introduction) I'd like you to keep time for us: OK?

Patient: Oh, I'm not sure ... how do you mean?

Counsellor: Well, this is very much **your** time. It's important that we use it carefully. I'll just check with you from time to time, how much time we have left, and how you want to use that time. OK?

Patient: Well, all right (hesitantly).

Counsellor: Let's see how it goes. How much time do we have left?

---

1. I am indebted to my colleague Dr Steve Baldwin for the suggestion of this technique.

Making introductions

Before beginning the formal 'business' it is appropriate for the counsellor to put his role in context. The patient may have arrived with specific expectations, based perhaps upon prior reading, or the shared experience of friends or family. Before beginning to 'work' on the problems the counsellor may choose to illustrate what he may offer, and what will be expected of the patient.

Counsellor: Before we begin properly let me clarify a few of the rules I have for myself. So far I know virtually nothing about you. You will tell me only what you choose to tell me. I'll respect everything that you say – I'll just take it at face value. I don't expect you to mislead me about anything. I won't expect you to tell me anything that you would rather keep to yourself for whatever reason. You will be the one doing most of the work. I see our relationship as being a bit like a partnership: Tim Rice and Andrew Lloyd Webber writing pop opera; each with their own part, but a lot of working together. If you feel that your problem is a bit of a mystery, maybe we'll be like Sherlock Holmes and Dr Watson, looking for clues, trying to unravel it. OK? The bad news is that you will be cast as Watson – he always gets the hard work to do.

(Note the careful use of humour early in the relationship. Note also the use of common partnership analogies to demystify the counselling process.)

Within this introduction the counsellor will negotiate audio-taping the sessions, to allow the patient to keep a record for further exploration in her own time (Ellis and Grieger, 1977). A special emphasis will be given also to the importance of negotiating assignments from the session, to allow 'learning in the real world'. Finally, the counsellor will suggest that a diary or daily log be used to promote the constructive reflection on life and the changes which it brings daily. Particular emphasis will be paid to recording thoughts/feelings (inaction) and behaviour (action). The aim of the assignments will be to promote the amount of action – choosing what needs to be done and doing it. The patient may be encouraged to notice how often her feelings appear to have no real relationship with what she is doing and vice versa. The aim is to change how she lives, not merely to tinker with her feelings.

The structure of the sessions

The counsellor aims to create an atmosphere of continuity of learning from one session to the next. Unlike 'treatments' which expose the person to highly technical or arcane procedures, here she is an active, equal collaborator. If she does not follow what is going on she will be encouraged to stop and ask, thereby increasing her understanding of the process.

The counsellor needs to take steps to enhance this style of counselling. The key feature will be the development of an agenda which will form the basis of the content of each session. The person is being encouraged to review how she 'constructs her own reality'. The counsellor aims to facilitate her making meaningful connections between her thoughts, feelings and events in her everyday life. To this end she will be encouraged to identify the content for each session; and to review at regular intervals, what she thinks of the session so far; what it means to her; and what (at the end of the session) any new-found perceptions might mean to her and her world.

Counsellor: What have you brought along today?
Patient: I'm still finding it difficult to mix with people ... you know, still avoiding things ... people I mean.
Counsellor: OK. Shall we work on this today? (nods) OK, anything else we need to include?

(Note that the counsellor begins at the point of entry into the session. Anything he might already know about the patient and identified 'problems', for example from a referral letter, is discounted in favour of what the person has 'brought with her'.)

Time

It is a convention in most counselling circles to allocate, in advance a predetermined number of sessions, each of a pre-set length. The reader may care to consider the wisdom of fixing the length or intervals between sessions. Many people in counselling tend to reify the 'golden hour', assuming that magical things happen during this time; many report spending much of the week waiting on the next appointment. The counsellor is aiming to encourage the person to recognize that each week there are 168 hours within which she has an opportunity to act, at each and every moment. The time spent with the counsellor should be perceived as no more than a reflection, or anticipation, of those lived moments.

Although some agreement about the (general) length of session was achieved at the outset, sessions may be curtailed by either party; especially when an important 'realization' has occurred; and the patient might be encouraged to 'go out and continue working on this'. Similarly, rather than abide by a fixed sessional arrangement, the counsellor might invite the patient to make the next appointment when an assignment has been completed. This arrangement reinforces the 'real' nature of the assignments. (Some patients never return for the next session. Whether this means that assignments were uncompleted, or that they simply chose not to proceed with more counselling, is open to question. Either way, it may be assumed that the person no longer needed the counsellor.)

Counsellor: Let's stop here. You've described how you **think** that you should deal with your son. You've reviewed the possible gains for making this change. Maybe what needs to happen now is for you to take this conviction away with you – for it certainly sounds like a conviction – and start changing that relationship with your son. What do you think that you will do first? No, wait, I'm getting ahead of myself. Maybe you should just go and **do it**! You can tell me what you did first, and what happened next, and so on, when we next meet. Let me leave it to you this time. Call me when you are ready to report on things. We can fix an appointment on the 'phone. OK?

(Note the counsellor's use of reflection: modelling changing his mind. Note also his acknowledgement of the patient's discovery of a 'conviction'.)

The counsellor can assume (correctly) that the patient will do something different with her son. More importantly, the patient has been given a clear message that she will do this (and likely more). Although it is a convention to describe this as an 'empowering' counselling strategy, I take the view that the person already has this power to do what needs to be done. The counsellor has merely acknowledged this. This might be called a 'validation' of the obvious.

The practice needs

These four principles involve eight counselling needs. These help shape the helping relationship, providing a skeleton upon which the change process might be established.

1. The need for structure

Many forms of counselling assume that the patient has some obligation to respond to the counselling process. If not, she must be 'blocking' in some way the counsellor's efforts. I would rather take the view that any failure to achieve the aims of counselling lies primarily with the counsellor. How the sessions are structured determines, to a great extent, what will emerge from the interaction. If the patient finds it difficult to articulate the nature of her difficulties, help her. If open-ended questions do not appear to help her clarify points, the counsellor needs to shift, temporarily, to closed questions.

Counsellor: You don' know how you feel about that? OK, let me ask, are you **satisfied** with how things are?

Patient: Well no.

Counsellor: Are you sure that you aren't satisfied?

Patient: Oh, yes, definitely! I'm not satisfied with me and Jimmy, and all that stuff … you know.

Counsellor: So you aren't satisfied. What does that mean for you?

Patient: Well, I guess I expected more from him. Its been a real let down the whole thing.

Counsellor: Let down? You feel disappointed?

Patient: Oh very disappointed.

Counsellor: OK. How do you deal with that disappointment?

2. The need for focus

The person is likely to bring a wealth of 'potential problems' to the session. One objective is to narrow the focus upon either what 'needs' to be addressed, or 'can be' dealt with now. The emphasis is upon helping the person to tease out her problems, distinguishing the various threads which contribute to the complexity of her life problems. Counselling is a sensitive form of psychological education: helping the person become aware of the different facets of a generalized problem; attaching useful descriptive labels to these parts of her overall functioning. Unlike some other forms of counselling, which emphasize the emotional resolution of the 'problem' the focus here is on the person's existing resources which she uses (perhaps unwittingly) to deal with the problem. The counsellor focuses most of his attention upon helping the person become more aware of these 'hidden assets'.

3. The need for 'nowness'

It is important to encourage the process of reflection, which will be central to the counselling process, as early as possible. There is no need to build up a broad picture of the patient, family, work or leisure context. It is assumed that the person will be ready to begin the process of change when, and only when, she is ready. Some readers may think that this is sacrilegious – abdicating a traditional faith in 'full assessment'; or fool-hardy – not allowing the counsellor to establish what, exactly, is being taken on. A principal assumption of the approach described here is that people are so enmeshed in the unwitting practice of 'everyday change' that establishing where, exactly, they are at any particular point is both impossible and unnecessary. The aim of the counselling process is to draw the person's attention to the inevitability of change; its everyday nature; and, most importantly, to the illusion of stability – especially of problems.

Where people are counselled on a formal basis, by appointment, the letter of introduction or the preparatory meeting might include the following 'awareness' message, as a scene-setter for the first formal appointment.

> '... perhaps I could ask you to give some thought to your problem. What is troubling you and what needs to be done to resolve it? You might also think about the changes, in your problem, which you have noticed recently. What have you noticed, which is different; which is in any way "out of the ordinary" for you? We shall discuss these when we meet.'

The intention here is to encourage the person to become aware of (a) her own problem; (b) what she believes is needed to solve it; and (c) what changes are occurring, naturally, as part of her everyday life. If the counsellor has any potential to 'promote' change, it lies here in the facilitation of the person's awareness of her 'natural' change processes.

4. The need for development

Counselling aims to help the person add to her 'learning from experience'. The counsellor's objectives are to help her appreciate how she constructs her emotional reality, and how she might acquire alternative ways of dealing 'constructively' with difficult life events. The emphasis is upon learning how to cope with life in general. Experimentation with specific life problems, or even with specific 'cognitive processes' like manipulation of memories, fantasies or current experiences, can contribute much to this reconstruction process.

Many therapies aim to encourage acceptance. This has a place here: helping the patient to distinguish between what can and cannot be changed. Many people who need counselling have been 'injured' by experiences of physical or psychological trauma; where the hurt is applied from the outside. Others have experienced loss – when someone or something is removed from their world, through death, divorce, separation, or redundancy. The 'trick' of living in such an incomplete or hostile world involves a similar kind of acceptance. It may be helpful to draw the person's attention to the timelessness of her 'wondering' about her problems: people have been considering how to deal with such losses, hurts and associated feelings for centuries. If the patient appears to believe that her experience of emotional hurt is in any way peculiar, the counsellor might suggest, as an assignment, reading a passage from the Bible, Koran, Shakespeare, etc. as a 'meditation' upon a time-honoured issue. The following is an example from Buddhist literature:

> What has been neglected cannot be restored
> immediately.
> Ills that have been accumulating for a long time
> cannot be cleared away immediately.
> One cannot enjoy oneself forever.

> Human emotions cannot be just right.
> Calamity cannot be avoided by trying to run
> away from it.
>
> (Cleary)

5. The need for experience

This approach to counselling emphasizes the person's experience of herself. The counselling session achieves nothing if it does not raise the person's awareness of how she constructs her experience of herself. Reflection alone is assumed to contribute little or nothing to change, other than as a preliminary to choosing alternative courses of action.

Counsellor: So what do you think of that?
Patient: Think? Oh, I dunno ... I just made a fool of myself.
Counsellor: How did you do that?
Patient: Well I did, didn't I? Everybody must have thought I behaved like a real jerk.
Counsellor: People said that? What exactly did they say?
Patient: Well ... they didn't exactly ... but I felt that they thought that ... about me ... I mean.
Counsellor: What are you saying ... you thought that they thought?
Patient: Well they were bound to ... weren't they?
Counsellor: Bound by what exactly?
Patient: Oh I dunno ... I just felt they would ... did I mean.
Counsellor: Yes, I'm sure you don't. For that reason I suspect that the next time you begin to make judgements about yourself, you will stop and wonder – just like you are doing now. When you leave here this afternoon, notice the first person you meet: any person, it doesn't matter. Ask yourself, how you can ever know what they think of you, if they don't actually tell you. Then ask yourself, what matters most, what they think of you, or what you think of yourself? You can give me the answers when next we meet.

6. The need for collaboration

The working alliance (Bordin, 1976) referred to here has a special meaning. The counsellor does not believe that he or she knows anything of worth about the person or her problem.

Certainly, there is no assumption that any theoretical explanation of distress or mental health has any relevance to this personal inquiry. Instead there is an emphasis upon partnership and guided discovery: both parties will learn something from the exploration, which previously may only have been glimpsed, 'through a glass darkly'. I make no apologies for suggesting that the relationship here might be more akin to that of athlete and sports coach: the person needs to develop some aspect of herself – this does not represent all of herself, or even, necessarily, the most important parts. The counsellor offers support and feedback, as appropriate – guiding the person's exploration of her problems, focusing upon what needs to be done now.

7. The need for holism

The counsellor assumes that the person's actions (behaviour) thinking and feelings are largely inseparable from one another. More importantly, he assumes that people choose not only actions, but also thoughts and feelings. The patient who describes feeling 'guilty' may be asked to describe what exactly they are doing to effect this. The counsellor attempts to draw relationships between the way a person exercises control over thoughts, feelings and actions. These are not distinct from one another, they only appear to be so. The use of simple questions, which appear on first hearing to be ridiculous (or provocative), may sensitize the person to the complex wholeness of her experiences. The counsellor encourages the person to explore the possibility that all of her experiences – of her thoughts, feelings and actions – are interlinked, all part of a total experience.

Patient: It's awful. I just feel so guilty all the time.
Counsellor: How do you do that?
Patient: Do what?
Counsellor: Feel guilty all the time.
Patient: (in a loud voice) I don't know. It just happens to be so.
Counsellor: Didn't we agree that nothing just happens? Do you feel guilty right now.
Patient: I'm not sure. I was mad at you for saying that.
Counsellor: Are you sure? You felt 'mad' but not 'guilty'? How did you do that, then? Feel 'mad' I mean. You raised your voice, uh huh?

Patient: I guess I did. Sorry.

Counsellor: What else were you doing? What was going on in your head? Can you recall?

Patient: I just thought … who does he think he is, he's … oh, I could have hit you.

Counsellor: But you didn't. How did you do that … choose not to hit me I mean?

(Note the counsellor's interest in the patient's thinking and pursuit of the patient's 'explanation' of which, at first, she is unaware.)

8. The need for flexibility

The counselling approach described briefly here is unashamedly eclectic: a small number of core assumptions about human experience serve as the basis for embellishment with any one of a number of counselling methods drawn from a whole range of schools of thought. The sophistication of the approach lies in the counsellor's choice of technique. As Lueger and Sheikh (1989) observed:

> Accused of theoretical sloppishness, if not contradiction, the eclectic therapist is likely to take satisfaction and confidence from the precision of the technique-to-problem fit … contrary to common sense and conventional wisdom, different therapies are not more effective with different problems.

Although scientific purists may be upset, much is to be gained from employing an eclectic, trans-theoretical approach. People make changes in their lives for a multiplicity of reasons. The reader might care to ask what part, if any, the following have played in shaping the conditions which resulted in making a choice regarding a specific course of action:

- a chance encounter with a friend or stranger
- a traumatic accident, to yourself or others
- a serious illness
- reading a book, poem, newspaper or magazine article
- seeing a film or viewing a work of art
- hearing familiar or new pieces of music
- recalling the past

- contemplating the present
- imagining the future
- looking in a mirror

This very limited list might serve as the basis for reminding the counsellor of the kind of events which change the course of people's lives. Indeed, these are likely to be examples of more potent factors than any so-called therapeutic techniques. The counsellor may select techniques which in some way mirror the influences from the everyday world. If the patient continues to follow her 'traditional' patterns of behaviour, she is likely to maintain her problem. The counsellor aims to help her notice how even everyday events – like looking in a mirror – are part of an ongoing reflection process, tied to the changing nature of her life. Possession of this awareness is a vital part of the empowering process of counselling.

Conclusion

This chapter has provided an overview of some of the issues involved in counselling for behaviour change. The author assumes that change in the patient's behaviour precedes the change in her self-concept, or any other notion of 'selfhood'. People change the way they think about themselves after they have made some change – however small – in their behaviour. Given this assumption, the counsellor focuses attention on how the person thinks about herself, and how such thinking might provide a link to her behaviour, outside the counselling scenario. To a large extent, the counsellor is curious about the way the person constructs 'feelings' but is largely disinterested in examining these emotional responses direct. Feelings are assumed to be a 'spin off' from the fuller lived-experience of the person, evidenced by her activity in the world.

3

Genetic Counselling

Allison J. Williams

It comes as a surprise to many people that nurses are employed in the traditionally scientific and medical field of genetics (Williams, 1994). However, if nurses are considered to be exemplary communicators, then given the integral components of genetic counselling as a helping and facilitating process, they have a valuable role to play in delivering such a service. Historically, genetics has had an image of being removed from mainstream medicine and therefore little attention has been paid to the lessons learned from such a model of service delivery in terms of application to other areas of medical, and more recently, nursing practice. Confusion has also existed surrounding the relationship between genetics and eugenics and this must be addressed. By definition, genetics is the study of inheritance whereas eugenics is the science that deals with all influences that improve the inborn quality of the human race, particularly through the control of hereditary factors. Genetics services are not associated with eugenics, the most extreme example of which was demonstrated in Nazi Germany. Genetics services are in the business of providing information and choice and are strongly opposed to the use of genetic tests or related measures to detect abnormalities purely on the basis that their detection can facilitate economic savings through any form of social control.

Genetics is currently one of the most rapidly developing areas of medicine and as such impinges on many allied health cares including general medicine, obstetrics, psychiatry, child health and surgery (particularly in the instance of inherited cancers). Primary care initiatives dictate that genetic screening may be devolved in the future and it is not unrealistic to expect that genetic factors and technology will impact on almost all nurses within the next decade. It is therefore imperative that we dispel the myths surrounding genetics and prepare for the scientific and client-centred culture that will inevitably ensue.

Individuals and families may be referred to the service for various different reasons, all of which will create a counselling need. The level of intervention will in part be defined by the reason for referral and the access mechanism to the service. Referrals may be received as a result of a child being born, unexpectedly, with a possibly inherited disorder, or of a prenatal screening test detecting an anomaly resulting in the need for further information, and potentially, reproductive choice. Such situations call for immediate counselling response, especially as the issue of genetic disease is often brand new to the family. Individuals seeking genetic counselling as a result of a known family history may have anticipatory knowledge of risks to themselves and future generations and the counselling focus is likely to be different. Assumptions must never be made concerning the level of knowledge and of anxiety that individuals in any of these circumstances experience. It is possible that the counselling needs of the known group of clients can be greater than in the crisis response group given that previous family experiences and myths need also to be addressed.

Genetics is an exciting and challenging field in which to work as a nurse. This chapter aims to identify common areas of counselling practice applicable to all aspects of nursing and to outline issues and experiences unique to this specialist field at the moment but which may become generally more applicable in the not too distant future.

Communication or counselling?

Much research has been undertaken in recent years outlining the essential need for communication within nursing practice. Research in the late 1960s clearly demonstrated that patients complain more about lack of information than any other aspect of their medical and nursing treatment (Cartwright, 1964; Raphael, 1969). The classic studies of the relationship between information, pain, anxiety and stress reinforced the need for communication in holistic patient care (Hayward, 1975; Boore, 1978), and on this basis, the focus on the theory of communication and skills training has been evident within nurse education in recent years. The term 'communication' has however become somewhat outdated with the advent of the buzz word 'counselling'. This is neither a new word nor a new practice but has almost been adopted by writers and researchers in the last two decades and described as a development in people management.

Tschudin (1991) states that to describe counselling is as difficult as to describe the essence of nursing itself and that the term is used in many and varied ways. This concept is clearly demonstrated in 1990s' society where connotations associated with the term are extensive; even a visit to the bank manager to discuss your overdraft may now be termed 'financial counselling'. The British Association of Counselling (BAC) describes the task of counselling as giving the client an opportunity to explore, discover and clarify ways of living more satisfying and resourcefully which could possibly be loosely associated with money management but can more realistically be applied to dealing with people in their roles as receivers of health care.

One of the unfortunate misconceptions of counselling is that it can imply an inability to cope with a situation and this is a notion that needs to be dispelled for both patients and nurses to become comfortable with the practice, particularly within genetics as the emotional and information issues involved are often unique to this area.

If counselling is associated with psychotherapy then it is rarely used within nursing and requires extensive skills and training. If, however, it is described as both a relationship and a process which involves a repertoire of skills emphasizing self-help and choice, then it is not an extension of the communication process we have all grown up with in our dealings with patients? Nurses are often comfortable with the concept of communicating but may be afraid of the seemingly unknown entity of counselling. I would argue that very few nurses are counsellors per se but that the majority of nurses use counselling skills everyday and we must reflect on the application of this practice.

The use of counselling in genetic nursing practice

In order to identify and discuss counselling practice within the role of a genetic nurse, it is necessary to describe first what genetic counselling involves and the role nurses play in this service.

> Genetic counselling is the process by which
> patients or relatives at risk of a disorder which
> may be hereditary are advised of the
> consequences of the disorder, the probability of
> developing or transmitting it and of the ways in
> which this may be prevented or ameliorated.
>
> (Harper)

It is a communication process dealing with the human problems associated with the occurrence, or the risk of occurrence of a genetic disorder in a family and involves facilitating individuals to understand the associated medical facts and make informed choices about their own actions. Adjustment to the disorder in a family member and/or to the risk of recurrence of that disorder is an equally important focus of genetic counselling. The process can therefore be defined as comprising three equally important integral components:

- diagnosis
- risk estimation
- counselling support

All aspects of the process are associated with the gathering and giving of information to empower clients to make their own informed choices. The BAC definition of counselling makes no mention of the role of information and therefore it could be questioned that the term 'genetic counselling' is indeed misleading and in fact the process is more aptly described as an information service which utilizes advanced counselling skills in communicating with patients.

The role of the genetics nurse depends in part on the focus of the genetics service in which he/she is employed. Many services could be described as 'nurse-led' with initial contact and definition of the genetic counselling contract taking place between the nurse and client at home. A model of pre-clinic home visiting, as adopted by some services, has many advantages, the first being to establish the family understanding of the purpose and reason for their referral. Counselling should always be at the request of the client, and no one can properly be 'sent' for counselling. Frequently genetics referrals are instigated without prior discussion with the family who may then be anxious or even resistant to the prospect of being part of a service for which they have little prior knowledge and understanding (the image of genetics amongst the general population is still one of mystique). It may be that the referred individual/family has no concerns or worries and that it is the referring doctor who is asking the questions. Genetics is a client-centred service and should take account of this and the genetic counselling process may therefore not progress beyond this initial contact. The collection of relevant information, drawing up a family pedigree and identification of other family members from whom information may be required will form part of the agenda for this initial contact although in practice, it may be that existing barriers will need to be broken down over a period of several sessions before this is possible. Ultimately the aim will be to prepare families for the clinic appointment where they are likely to receive clinical information and diagnosis if available. The nurse will have invested time in facilitating definition of family questions to be addressed during their genetic counselling appointment and these will set the agenda for that encounter. The purpose of this measure is to ensure not only that their questions are answered if possible, but that the questions which have no answers can also be addressed. Such a model also aims to ensure that clients do not receive information that they have specifically requested that they do not want. The nurse will attend the clinic appointment with the family as their advocate to ensure that their agenda is adhered to and to enable them to then contract with the family for the follow-up counselling support they need thereafter.

Genetics literature places great emphasis on clinical/scientific diagnosis and risk estimation. Whilst an integral part of the genetics counselling process, this information purely facilitates inevitable decision-making on the part of the genetics patient and in reality, given the fact that most genetic disorders are individually rare, it is not uncommon to be counselling families where there is no firm clinical data. Harper (1993) states that contrary to much medical practice where doctors may give directive advice to patients on the basis of clinical information and results, the practice of most geneticists and genetic nurses is one of non-directive counselling. Clarke (1994) poses the question 'is non-directive genetic counselling possible?' and it can be argued that whilst practitioners may aspire to this end, in reality it is impossible to ignore completely personal socialization and prejudice when participating in any counselling relationship. Self awareness and the ability to deal with personal bias outside the counselling session is a vital attribute of a good counsellor. There will always be instances where we do not believe that the right decision has been made, but from whose perspective are we making that judgement? If we believe in non-directive counselling, that discomfort belongs to the counsellor and is one which needs to be addressed outside the counselling relationship through supervision.

Non-directiveness may in some instances be perceived by the counsellee as being particularly unhelpful, especially within the realm of reproductive decision-making where time for reflection is likely to be limited and couples may actively seek advice rather than facilitation. It is possible that their experience of health care services up to this point has been within a directive medical model and therefore they are battling not only with the decision at hand but also with the unfamiliar management context within which it is being handled. The questions 'What do you think we should do?' and 'What would you do if you were in our place?' are frequently asked and the genetic nurse needs to feel comfortable with not feeling pressured to provide answers but to facilitate exploration and reflection to help individuals to arrive at their own decision. Anger may be frequently expressed at this time and may be targeted at the counsellor as he/she can often be perceived as the 'bad guy' who refuses to help and advise. It must also be recognized that many of the issues concerned will present ethical dilemmas to both counsellor and counsellee, especially within the realm of termination of pregnancy and exploration of ethical stance may play a big part in decision-making.

Harper (1993) stresses that it is not the duty of a doctor to order the lives of others but to ensure that individuals have the facts to enable them to make their own decisions. This concept of informed choice features prominently in both nursing and medical literature and within the context of genetics, it is generally accepted that whilst non-directive counselling philosophy dictates that counsellors cannot take responsibility for the decisions their clients make, there is a clear need to ensure that information is given in an unbiased way and at a level appropriate for client understanding and assimilation. This requires a level of skill and knowledge on the part of the practitioner such that the same information can be given in many and varied ways taking account of language and academic barriers. Harper (1993) acknowledges that mis-interpretation of facts is not uncommon in genetic counselling which reinforces the need for clear, unbiased information. When discussing recurrence risks for a recessive condition for example, the explanation can be offered in many ways:

- 'There is a 1 in 4 risk of recurrence'.
- 'There are 3 out of 4 chances that the baby will be fine'.
- 'There is a 25% chance that the baby will be affected'.
- 'There is a 75% chance that the baby will not inherit the problem'.

In mathematical terms, all the above statements mean exactly the same, but each can individually sound very different. It is therefore imperative that as many different formats are used when giving such information so that the client can select his/her own perspective upon which to base the resultant decision. Another feature of decision-making within genetic counselling is that individuals themselves and other family members may be required to make the same decisions over and over again with successive pregnancies and generations. It is important to acknowledge the fact that clients need to feel comfortable that any choice they make is the right one for them at that moment in time in the particular circumstances they find themselves. This acceptance is particularly signifi-cant given that faced with the same decision again at a different point in their lives, any subsequent choice may be different. Indeed, in the experience of the author, inconsistent decision-making is commonplace and if not carefully facili-tated can lead to feelings of guilt and anger concerning previous choices thus reinforcing the need for a non-directive approach.

Models and skills for counselling in genetics

Genetic counselling does not ascribe to any one particular model of counselling and in practice may be a hybrid of many different styles depending on the counselling, the needs of any particular individual and the situation at hand. As Tschudin (1991) states, 'ideally we should dispense with all models and use only ourselves, our own humanity, to help a person'. However, using a model as a framework for the helping process often facilitates definition of the counselling contract. The Rogerian model of non-directive, client-centred counselling most closely reflects the aim of genetic counselling. Egan's problem management model, whilst describing a non-directive approach to facilitate change implies a more proactive approach to problem solving which may be relevant to certain genetic counselling situations but which bears less relevance to areas where clients are adjusting to the inevitable with no choices to make or actions to take. Unlike many counselling relationships, the ascertainment and giving of information is integral to the genetic counselling process. Therefore the focus, rather than being on the model in question, should concern the listening and questioning skills involved.

Egan describes the concept of helping clients tell their stories and this aptly reflects the information ascertainment phase of genetic counselling in addition to the ongoing supportive process. The accuracy and content of the genetic client's story is imperative as it is the basis for all future events. The content of the story is defined by the client in the sense that they control personal disclosure but can be equally reliant on other family members for information. The questioning skills of the counsellor and the counselling relationship itself can significantly influence the level of disclosure and therefore the success of the genetic counselling process in this context. The relationship and counselling environment must inspire confidence in the client such that they feel in control of disclosure and do not feel that they will be judged in the process. In support of this philosophy the majority of genetic nurse–client interactions take place in the home. Security is particularly pertinent when obtaining a family history to draw up a pedigree – one of the major tools for genetic counselling. Issues of consanguinity, marital status, non-paternity or unknown paternity are vital when establishing inheritance patterns but may have never been openly discussed in the family and create potential for considerable tension and distress. Closed questioning and judgemental non-verbal communication within such a process will have a deleterious effect. The use of open questioning is therefore employed as much as possible in order to leave the client free to respond as they would wish. Such questioning inevitably means that the process is much longer and results in information being disclosed which is not necessarily relevant to the issue in question but which may be pertinent to the assessment of family dynamics and the emotional state of the counsellee. This is interspersed with affective questioning approaches to encourage exploration and discussion of feelings and attitudes. Open questioning, whilst allowing clients to tell their own stories, also provides the opportunity for the counsellor to observe and actively listen to what is truly being said. Listening to verbal and non-verbal responses will facilitate reflective dialogue to ensure correct interpretation and set the scene for effective probing if appropriate. Active listening involves actually hearing what is being said and this includes the emotional context of the interaction. Genetics rarely deals with situations requiring immediate response and action, therefore knowing when to stop asking questions and temporarily withdraw from the situation is vital to protect the long-term relationship with, and integrity of, the counsellee.

Tschudin (1991) describes varying stages of counselling acknowledging the fact that a neat linear progression from identifying the problem to adjustment is unrealistic. Certainly within genetics a cyclical approach is a more accurate representation of the counselling process – cyclical in the sense that a file is never closed on a family and reactivation after varying periods of no support is defined by life events, reproduction, subsequent generations asking questions and scientific advances. Reactivation may be inspired by a different perspective on an existing problem or the occurrence of newly identified problems relating to the family condition. The fact that an individual has had counselling previously does not directly correspond with the amount of help they need on subsequent occasions and old experiences inevitably surface in any new counselling episode. Because of the nature of genetic disease, the counselling inevitably encompasses not only index cases but also additional family members, therefore relying on the counsellor to have an understanding of family life and dynamics.

Street (1994) states that families need to cope with the daily problems of living, to face up to the challenges of development and to provide for the needs of their members. The mechanism by which this is achieved depends upon clear roles and relationships within the family unit and the ability to identify and build upon existing coping strategies. The diagnosis of an inherited condition and the subsequent investigations and enquiries that occur create the potential for disruption of existing family dynamics, an event that must be avoided at all costs. Norms of interactions based upon inclusion, control and intimacy can be destroyed by insensitive exploration. Family members may be dependent upon one another for information and the conflict between privacy and needing to ask a relative for help can cause untoward difficulties. Often information can only be obtained from previous generations and enquiry can frequently be misinterpreted as blame. Any information request is always directed through the index case to avoid individuals being approached by professionals without prior warning and explanation and codes of confidentiality must be strictly obeyed. The result of any family investigation often means that additional family members, who may or may not be at risk of the condition in question themselves, require counselling support for varying reasons including guilt, self blame and anger towards previous generations and unaffected family members. Relatives who have 'escaped' the family condition may often need support coming to terms with what can be described as survivor guilt and this can require as much adjustment as to the disease itself.

All of these individual counselling interactions may be occurring simultaneously and due to the service delivery mechanisms are likely to involve the same counsellor. If conflict is occurring within the family, the counsellor needs to clear about confidentiality boundaries for the situation to be tenable. Difficulties may occur as a result of information issues, where family members refuse to allow access to records and results. The counsellor may know the precise details him/herself because of separate interactions but cannot divulge this information. Hence all parties involved must be made aware of such dilemmas but reassured that their confidence will never be breached without prior agreement. Conflict may also arise as a result of differing rates of progression towards adjustment and the strategies employed. The issue is particularly noticeable within couples, where resentment that one partner seems to be coming to terms with the problem quicker than the other is often misinterpreted as uncaring. It is important in such instances, be they between couples or discrete family units, that the counsellor facilitates not only individual progress but also acknowledges the resultant relationship difficulties which may need to be dealt with separately to redress the family dynamic balance. This process cannot be subject to time constraints. Unlike many counselling relationships in nursing, genetic counselling is a continuum along which crisis counselling is interspersed with periods of little interaction and longer-term developmental type counselling and that from a referral of one individual, appropriate counselling contracts may be negotiated with numerous family members.

When dealing with families caution must be exercised to ensure delineation of the subject remit with which the counsellor is prepared to work. Frequently counselling needs which are unrelated to the purpose of the genetics interaction will be identified as a by-product of exploring individual and family problems. These may need to be subcontracted out to another counsellor with the client's agreement to protect the context of the genetic counselling relationship. There is often a fine balance between related and unrelated issues as genetic counselling can impinge on many life and relationship problems; careful exploration must therefore precede any separation of issues.

Genetic counselling scenarios

Applying the aforementioned principles to hands-on counselling experience in this field is dictated by the issue, disease, timing, personality and previous experiences of the individuals involved in the process. There is no standard genetic counselling session and neither should be there. However, there are issues and circumstances which could be loosely grouped together and rather than present any one interaction as a

transcribed event, the following scenarios aim to give an outline of the counselling needs which may be identified.

Scenario 1: Pre-conceptual counselling

Sarah and Daniel are both in their late twenties, unmarried but
in a stable relationship. They are planning to start a family next
year and approached their GP asking about the risks of cystic
fibrosis to their future children because Daniel has a nephew
affected with this condition. A direct referral was made for
genetic counselling and an evening home visit was arranged.
The context of the visit as defined by the couple was as follows:

Their information needs:	What exactly is Cystic Fibrosis? How is the condition inherited? Are all children equally handicapped by the condition? What are the risks to our children?
Their counselling needs:	• There was a fundamental difficulty between them concerning disclosure of family information and previous relationships.
	• Daniel does not believe in abortion under any circumstances and Sarah is adamant she does not want an affected child.
	• Daniel does not feel ready to start thinking about a family but Sarah feels desperate to get pregnant before she reaches 30.

There were three 2-hour counselling sessions with this couple
addressing their basic communication difficulties before
carrier testing could be undertaken. This was essential in
preparation for any decisions which may have to be made
should they both be CF carriers. It transpired that Daniel had a
previous partner who became pregnant and had a social

termination of pregnancy without telling him. He was carrying a lot of anger concerning this and had never told Sarah. Daniel was also feeling pressured by what he described as Sarah's biological clock and felt that they needed to be more financially secure before having a baby. The genetic counselling had facilitated discussion of all these concerns that they had been avoiding as a couple for months. Eventually they worked through these issues and compromised on the financial/biological clock issue by agreeing to put off starting a family for another year. They were clear that they both wanted carrier testing but would put off discussion of reproductive decision-making until they knew the results. It transpired that Daniel did not carry his family mutation and therefore their combined risk of having an affected child was significantly less than 1 per cent.

Scenario 2: Prenatal testing and diagnosis

Allison is 23 years old and pregnant for the first time. At 32 weeks gestation she has an ultrasound scan following complaints of abdominal pain. It is noted that the baby has bent femurs and Allison is informed by her obstetrician that her baby has osteogenesis imperfecta (brittle bones). She is alone in the clinic because her husband Keith is at work. She is so stunned by the news that she cannot ask questions and goes straight home. When Keith arrives home from work, he finds Allison in a very distressed state and they to back to the hospital. They are told that there are several forms of osteogensis, that it is believed that their child has a severe form of the condition for which there is no treatment and that termination of pregnancy would have been recommended if this was diagnosed earlier in pregnancy. They are told that elective caesarean section at 38 weeks' gestation will be the preferred form of delivery to minimize trauma to the baby. They are referred for genetic counselling five weeks following the birth of their daughter Lianne.

Their information needs:
- What is osteogenesis imperfecta?
- Is it hereditary? If so, whose fault is it that Lianne is affected?

- What is Lianne's prognosis? Will she ever walk? At this stage they were not able to think about further children.

Their counselling needs:
- Needed to address and deal with their anger towards their obstetrician for the way in which the bad news was broken.
- Allison was having tremendous difficulty bonding with Lianne.
- Her fears concerning handling her and possibly hurting her needed to be addressed. Allison was also afraid that Lianne was going to die and therefore didn't want to get too close.
- Blame – it is no-one's 'fault'.

The information available about the condition was able to assist in some of the counselling needs. Lianne has a mild form of osteogenesis; cuddles and nappy changes and any normal handling is not going to hurt her or put her at risk. Her condition is not life threatening and she will walk like other children. She will however be at greater risk of fractures through injury than her peers. It transpired after many counselling sessions and examinations that Keith also has the same condition. He has broken his leg five times in his life but does play competitive rugby! Allison has bonded very well with Lianne who is now three years old, very bright and fit and well. They have two more children, both with a different obstetrician to Lianne, both of whom are also affected with osteogenesis. In her subsequent pregnancies, Allison has controlled the scanning information herself and has had two normal vaginal deliveries following spontaneous onset of labour. When any new health professional meets Lianne and her brothers, varying levels of concern are raised. Allison deals with this herself being empowered with a high level of information and understanding about the family condition. It is not a problem for them as open access to support from their genetic nurse facilitates coping and early professional intervention if conflicts arise.

Scenario 3: Loss, bereavement and breaking bad news

Genetic counselling is often associated with loss which can take on many guises:

- Death – this may be a pregnancy loss or death of a child/family member.
- Pending death of self or a family member as a result of predictive testing.
- Loss of function due to onset or pending onset of disability.
- Loss of perception of self and role as a result of pending or actual disability.
- Loss of dreams for the future – this is often associated with reproduction and hopes and dreams of family life/children.
- Trying to accept that one's child will not have a 'normal' life.

Buckman (1984) states that any news that drastically and negatively alters the patient's view of her or his future is defined as 'bad news' and that the impact of this depends on the size of the gap between the patient's expectations (including his or her ambitions and plans) and the medical reality of the situation. On this basis, the genetic counselling interactions which deal with information preceding any sense of loss are synonymous with breaking bad news. Naturally, most people do not want to be told that they themselves, a relative or a future child are at risk of having or developing a disease. Similarly genetic counsellors do not want to be the bearers of such information but this is an integral part of the function of counselling in this area and must be addressed. Feelings of anxiety at breaking bad news are common even amongst the most experienced counsellors who will often admit to feeling inadequate in such situations. Given that this is such a difficult issue to deal with, and is probably the most central focus of all genetic counselling interactions, it is important to recognize social, personal and professional factors which can both hinder and help the counsellor and counsellee. Buckman (1992) states that since our society values the sick less than the healthy, discussions of ill-health implicitly carry overtones of social demotion. This is particularly pertinent when discussing a late-onset genetic condition with a patient and may need to be both acknowledged and discussed within the concept of self-perception and is part of the adjustment process as implicit in the definition of genetic counselling previously outlined.

Making assumptions about people's reactions to such news is dangerous and as Buckman says 'there is only one safe assumption – it's not safe to assume anything!' Anticipating reactions and planning interactions accordingly is likely to have an adverse effect on the process. Acknowledging our own feelings and overcoming the fear that the messenger will be blamed for the bad news is essential. As health care professionals we must never forget that we are also human beings and when dealing with people in distress, we cannot abandon our human feelings. When you have to tell a couple that the baby they are carrying has a life-threatening condition, I would challenge any nurse that claimed to feel nothing. In genetics, it is possible that this may be the third or fourth time you have had to break this exact same bad news to the same couple and you inevitably share in their distress. We must acknowledge that it is not unacceptable to display our emotions in front of our clients provided it is in a controlled way and the focus of empathy and the dynamics of the counselling relationship are not altered.

It is generally accepted that loss associated with death is accompanied by bereavement but any type of loss should be credited with similar experiences. Kubler-Ross (1970) describes the bereavement process associated with death as comprising stages of denial, anger, bargaining, depression, acceptance and finally hope. These features can equally be identified in the process of coping with any form of loss. The misconception of a linear progression through these phases is borne out by Buckman (1992) who identifies a more simplified three-stage model, acknowledging that each individual expresses emotions that are characteristic of that person, not the stage, and that several emotions may be expressed simultaneously. Patients who have lost a pregnancy often express distress that after a very short time, family and friends expect them to have adjusted to their loss. Comments such as 'you should have got over this by now' and 'well, it wasn't as if you knew the baby and then it died' are perceived as devaluing their loss and only serve to extend their grief and period of adjustment. Loss is a very personal concept and therefore reactions to different forms of loss will vary enormously between individuals. Sylvia, a woman with 10 children who had a still birth at age 40 was told by a younger female relative who had recently miscarried her first child that their grief was incomparable and that she should be grateful that she had 10 children and count her blessings. Sylvia was devastated by this reaction which was repeated by many friends and relatives. In counselling she expressed an acute sense of loss associated with not only the baby but the infant, toddler, child and adult that individual would have grown into – she was mourning the loss of all these people and she saw her deceased baby as being not just the eleventh child. One should never underestimate the extent of the counsellee's feelings and grief.

Conclusion

Genetic counselling is a complex combination of interactions with people who are seeking information about risks of genetic disease to themselves, relatives or future children. It is not counselling within the strictest definitions but is more a communication process which involves the use of advanced listening, attending and questioning skills. Interactions are often associated with breaking bad news and coping with loss.

Whilst similar to many other areas of counselling within nursing practice, the unique feature of Genetic Counselling must be the relationship with family dynamics and the fact that in addition to 'bad news' the nature of genetic disease means that often we are giving people information that could be more aptly described as 'ambiguous news'. Whether the information contained in any genetic counselling episode is good, bad, or ambiguous, some form of decision-making is likely to ensue and it is this decision-making process which often produces the greatest counselling demand. The helping process should take the form of non-directive counselling and this is often perceived by the counsellee as being unhelpful especially when dealing with uncertainties. If the essence of genetic counselling is the counsellor's ability to transmit genetic information about an inherited disorder of concern to the counsellee so that it will be incorporated into decision-making (Emergy and Pullen, 1984), then the emotional needs of the individual and family could be perceived as secondary to their need for information stemming from genetic probabilities and diagnosis. However, there is an implicit responsibility for genetic counsellors to address emotional factors and facilitate adaptation of existing coping mechanisms. Accepting that as nurses we don't have to 'do' anything within such interactions is often the hardest lesson to learn. The act of listening is often all we can offer but we should never underestimate the difficulty or the impact of this seemingly simple task. Preparing for listening, creating an appropriate environment and giving someone time demonstrates that you value their needs but actually hearing what is said is the essence of good counselling practice.

As genetics moves out of the specialist arena into more general areas of nursing and medical practice, the concept of holistic patient care will need to be extended to encompass factors of inheritance and family. This will require modification of current care planning and delivery philosophies such that we consider the impact of diagnosis and management on the counselling needs of patients and potentially at-risk relatives.

The adage 'first do no harm' rarely has such psychological implications as when dealing with and preserving family dynamics and coping strategies. Within the context of genetics, we may never have all the answers to all the questions but I would argue that this is how it should be. Our role is to help people to find their own answers through effective counselling and to live with the consequences.

4

Counselling Children

Jim Richardson

Introduction

The counselling of children is a highly complex domain, the practice of which requires a range of specialist insights and skills. On occasion, it will be necessary to refer children and their families to a children's counsellor. It is important that the children's nurse recognizes the situation which requires such a referral. However, it is likely that in the paediatric nurse's daily work all communication with the children contains an element of counselling. For this reason a careful consideration of the factors which affect communication with children will allow the nurse to take a more systematic approach to talking with children. This will promote mutual understanding between nurse and child and should make communication more effective and satisfying.

It is useful to consider exactly what the word 'counselling' might mean in the context of working with children. Burnard (1992) suggests that counselling is a relationship between people in which the focus of purposeful conversation is on issues of interest or concern to the person counselled. This relationship is fuelled by the wish of the counsellor to help the person counselled to achieve the insights which will help this person to understand their own situation and act in their own interest. Of course, these are many considerations to be taken into account when working with children which will influence the course of talking with children. Crompton (1992) recounts how nurses in one children's unit preferred not to use the term 'counselling' since they felt it was a jargon term with an imprecise meaning which tended to be misunderstood. These nurses preferred to talk about 'looking, learning and listening' when trying to express the counselling component of their work. Crompton herself emphasizes that she sees counselling activity as being comforting and reassuring by reinforcing children's own skills and resources to cope with difficulties. Taken together these ideas seem to provide an understandable definition for 'counselling'.

Hilton Davis (1993) summarizes the characteristics of counselling as:

- 'Respecting the individual's freedom to choose as they themselves see fit.
- Facilitation of the individual's own decision-making.
- Encouragement of the individual's own effectiveness.
- Careful exploration of the situation/problem from the viewpoint of the person seeking help.
- Agreement of aims, and negotiation as necessary.
- Provision of relevant information, if possible, in ways that are clear and effective.'

In the work of the children's nurse the child patient may face many difficulties; enduring and adapting to illness, preparing for and understanding medical treatment and accepting the necessity of that treatment. When the nurse's thoughtful communication is geared towards helping the child and his or her family cope with the challenges facing them, this can be seen as counselling. When working with children it is important to appreciate that children of different stages of cognitive development may have particular difficulty in understanding complex situations. As a consequence, simple counselling activity with children will probably involve more information giving than would normally be expected when working with adults. The nurse in this respect might be seen as an interpreter.

In communicating with children it will be particularly significant to strive to understand the child's conception of the situation and related events. This emphasizes the reciprocal nature of purposeful communication between child and nurse. Effective communication can only be framed when the nurse has explored the child's viewpoint and found the messages which will be relevant and helpful for the child. This in turn will allow the format in which these messages should be offered to be established. This process involves talking to and listening to the child and constantly checking that meanings are understood. An open dialogue has to be established and this in itself requires that the nurse understand those factors which will help the child talk to the nurse. Equally important, of course, will be those factors which might hamper communication between nurse and child. The aim will be to create a situation in which the child feels free to express thoughts and feelings which the nurse is then in a position to understand.

The traditional route of counselling for adults has emphasized a conversational clarifying process which allows the person counselled to define what the problems or difficulties actually are. The following stage is for that person then to discern, in talking with the counsellor, which of his own abilities and coping strategies are most likely to help him to improve his situation. This process also allows the person counselled to identify unhelpful reactions and adaptations which prevent the situation being improved. It seems logical that such an approach could be helpful when working with children too.

Talking with children

Society's conception of what a child is, is constantly evolving. We are moving from thinking of children as small, under-developed adults with a limited capacity for realistic understanding to the point where children are now acknowledged as thinking, feeling, dynamically developing and unique individuals. Children are, however, different from adults and an appreciation of these differences is an important prerequisite for understanding the responses of children.

The development of thinking in childhood

Children's capacity for understanding and expressing that understanding is highly dependent on their stage of cognitive development and previous life experience. Meeting a new experience for the first time may stretch a child's capacity to interpret the meaning and significance of that experience. Without some insight into the process of cognitive development the conclusions which a child reaches based on immature reasoning may be very unexpected from an adult's point of view. The process of interpreting the world around us and how that process changes as we change from child to adult has long been a subject of interest to developmental psychologists. Development in children's ability to think and reason might be seen as a series of stages, such as that proposed by Piaget, in each of which the child develops a new constellation of skills. Cognitive development might also be seen as a process during which the child adds new abilities and insights to existing skills. The exact course of child cognitive development is still the source of much debate but is clearly a sequence which has certain common trends which can be discerned in all children. The work of the Swiss developmental psychologist Piaget provides an interesting framework for considering the developmental progress of children. Piaget was important in that he acknowledged the active participation of the child in his/her own development. He suggested that children construct their own reality through interacting with their environment and suggested several processes through which children use new information they gain from their experiences with the world:

- Assimilation – this is the process of absorbing new information received through the senses.
- Accommodation – the information assimilated is then manipulated so that it makes sense when compared with what the child has already learned and knows. In this way the stock of the child's understanding is increased.
- Equilibration – the child always seeks to maintain a balance in understanding. New information must be organized so as to contribute to a logical, sensible understanding. Material which cannot be 'fitted into' an overall understanding may be rejected.

Piaget, in observing the development of his own children, suggested that children's cognitive development can be organized into four major stages:

- A sensorimotor stage which occurs from birth until roughly 2 years of age. This stage is characterized by unplanned responses to environmental stimuli. As the child develops the motor ability to interact with the environment in more complex ways the information the child receives becomes more complex. So too do the ways the child handles this new information. During this period the child 'decentres', begins to see himself as an independent being separate from others, especially his mother. The child has not the ability at this stage to represent objects with, for example, words.

- A preoperational stage which lasts broadly from 2 until 6 years of age. At this stage the child's thinking develops quickly. He develops the ability to use representations for actions so that he can think through actions as a means of testing them rather than actually performing these actions. The child tends to be self-centred in his thinking which is a limiting factor and is inclined to be concrete and simplistic in the interpretations he makes of experiences and the solutions and conclusions he reaches about these experiences.
- A concrete operational stage which lasts roughly from 6 until 12 years of age. This stage is characterized by the rapid development of logical thinking organized into operations or strategies of thinking such as trial and error approaches to problems. The child's perception is broader and takes more factors into account such as the perspective of other people involved in the same situation. This stage includes the development of reasoning ability. During this period in their development children will tend to use a direct, concrete approach to communication and subtleties may well be lost on them.
- A formal operational stage lasting from around 12 years of age into adulthood. This stage is characterized by the development of logical, systematic approaches to the solving of problems. Possibilities are identified and a hypothetico-deductive approach taken to identifying the most likely solution to a problem. The more flexible thinking of this stage, therefore, develops more abstract features.

This thumbnail sketch outlines one theorist's attempt to organize and classify the complicated developmental progress in children's thinking throughout childhood. Many workers have elaborated and developed these theories since Piaget first suggested them in the first half of this century. More detailed information about developmental theories can be found in textbooks such as Bee (1995).

Language

One example of development in which trends can be noted for which the underlying processes are still incompletely understood is language. Language allows us to express our thoughts and feelings and the reception of language enables us to understand other people. Observing the course of development of children's language demonstrates how first the sounds are mastered from simple vocalic sounds to complex consonant sounds. We can hear how simple words are used in isolation and then combined with others to form more sophisticated language. As the child grows and develops we notice how the child begins to use the rules of grammar to make language use more conventional but also to aid in the clarity of spoken messages. Language development has, in broad outline, common similarities between children; it appears as a linear progression. We know roughly when a child's language is around the stage of development to be expected at that child's chronological age. We also know, for that child, what the next likely stage of language development is. The development of language ability is easy to observe but there is also a wide range of normal in this area of development. Children show themselves to be individual in their language development. This may be influenced by internal factors such as the child's innate ability to learn language or the ability to hear normally. External factors affecting speech development include the experience of hearing language used by others and having the opportunity to practise the sounds and patterns of speech.

Communication between people is not solely determined by the use of language. The subtleties of non-verbal communication such as body language, and paralanguage such as stress, emphasis and rhythm of speech as well as features such as hesitancy are also important. The ability to understand, and indeed use, these more subtle forms of communication is also developed during childhood. The use of word play and irony for humorous effect is not developed until late in childhood. Children's jokes reveal a good deal about their stage of cognitive development.

It is clear, therefore, that a knowledge of the sequence of language development will be helpful to the nurse who is communicating with a child. This knowledge will have to be tempered, however, by an understanding of the individuality of language development. Initial communication between nurse and child will be something of a diagnostic process during which the nurse assesses that particular child's particular communication abilities. This is a vital stage in communicating with a child as it allows us access to the child's abilities and perspectives and also allows us to establish the level of language which will be most appropriate for use with that child.

There are many features of language which will have to be taken into account when talking with children. Obvious diffi-culties will arise if the nurse and child do not share a common language. Communication in this case may have to take place through a third person as an interpreter, parents or older sib-lings may fulfil this role. This situation is less than ideal since it contradicts the principle that the communicating, counselling process is one that occurs between two people. The introduc-tion of a third party and the process of translating from one language to another introduces the possibility of distortions of meaning occurring. Such a situation also makes it difficult to keep communication confidential and this may have an inhibit-ing effect. By far the best solution is to find a nurse who shares the child's home language.

The culture from which the child comes will have important consequences for communication between child and nurse. Culture in this context should be understood in its widest sense. That is, the beliefs, values and behaviour of a group of people which are learned in childhood from elders and which are modified by the environment in which that group finds itself. This definition indicates that culture as an idea does not simply concern ethnic or racial groups but also class, gender and age factors as well as regional origin. Culture defines how that child will communicate and also the expectations that the child will have of the people he/she meets. Culture may define that boys communicate in a more open manner than girls or it may dictate that children, 'are seen but not heard', which may discourage the child from communicating directly with a strange adult. Cultural factors will also determine how non-verbal communication is used so that cross-cultural interpreta-tions may be difficult to make. The child from a Chinese back-ground who averts her gaze when talking to an English nurse but who smiles all the time may lead the nurse to think that the child is shy but agreeing with what she is saying. In fact, she may be communicating no more than polite respect for this unfamiliar adult. While culture is a feature which must be considered in communicating with children, great care must be taken to avoid stereotyping. This sort of attribution of characteristics to a person based on what is felt to be common features of his/her perceived cultural group is a risky manoeuvre. It denies the individuality and uniqueness of people and is just as likely to be inaccurate. The only way to be clear about a person's cultural beliefs and behaviour is to ask that person about these issues.

A language barrier can occur as a result of factors rather less obvious than nurse and child speaking different languages. Regional dialects or class-bound forms of language and accents can hamper common understanding. The nurse with a strong Scottish accent or who uses cockney slang may be very difficult for a child from Wales to understand – and vice versa! Equally, it should be obvious that a professional jargon such as that often used by doctors and nurse can be difficult for a child to interpret. Nurses may use a word such as 'washout' to indicate a mild lavage rinsing procedure but what kind of images does that raise in a child's mind? In the same way, children may share the use of special words used within the family which constitute a sort of family 'shorthand' or private language. This private, family use of language often deals with intimate and common issues such as elimination. It may take the nurse a moment to realize that the small child who declares that he, 'wants to make a smell', actually wants to defecate!

All children are dependent to some extent on their families, particularly their parents or principal carers. In a situation which the child experiences as new, unfamiliar or frightening the child may be reluctant to communicate directly with an unfamiliar adult and may feel more comfortable communicating through a parent. When approaching a child a balance must be struck between addressing a parent–child group and speaking directly to the child concerned. This balance is informed by the careful evaluation of the child's communication needs and preferences. A fine distinction is drawn between approaching the child as an individual on the one hand and, on the other hand, as an enmeshed member of a supportive and protective family group.

The following example of a conversation between a nurse and a child illustrates some of the points that have been discussed so far. Fred, a six year old, is in hospital for the first time after falling out of a tree and fracturing his femur three days ago. He is talking to Geraldine, a young children's nurse.

Geraldine: Hello, my name's Geraldine. I'm your nurse today, Fred.

Fred: My name is Frederick.

Geraldine: Oh, I'm sorry, it says on your notes that you're called Fred.

Fred: Yes, Mummy and Daddy call me Fred but *you* must call me Frederick.

Geraldine: OK, Frederick. Have you any friends to play with here?

Fred: Yes, but my best friend is Pierre.

Geraldine: Is your best friend French?

Frederick: Don't be silly. Pierre's a hamster – he's from Syria.

Geraldine: (gathering her composure). Would you like to play a game with me now?

Fred: No, my leg hurts now.

Geraldine: I'll get you a tablet for your sore leg.

Fred: That's just daft! How can a tablet in my tummy help my leg?

(Geraldine explains and Frederick takes his tablet. Sometime later he says his leg does not hurt anymore but he looks uncomfortable and restless.)

Geraldine: You look uncomfortable. Do you want to have a wee?

Fred: (Looks puzzled) What's that?

Geraldine: You know, when you go to the toilet.

Fred: Oh, you mean make water?

Geraldine: Yes.

Fred: Then why don't you say so? I'm not a baby. Go away.

Some important factors to be taken into account when communicating with children

Listen to the child

What the child has to say may not be immediately understandable to an adult as the child struggles to find a means of expressing thoughts and feelings. This does not mean that the child has nothing of value to say. Jerrett and Evans (1986) in a research project which investigated how children expressed their experience of pain spoke with one child who expressed her pain as being like a 'sausage'! At first sight this is rather bizarre and certainly would be open to misinterpretation by an adult. Further discussion, however, revealed that the child was suffering from a hot, tense pain which the child could only describe as being like a sausage frying in a pan. Sometimes time, effort and creative leaps of logic are necessary to decipher children's messages.

Give the child time

It is natural that when the child struggles to express and describe unfamiliar experiences that time is necessary for this. It should be clear that to try to rush the child will serve to inhibit that child's attempts at communication.

Respect the child

A consciousness of children's rights will reflect that the child is a human being just like you, only younger. It is important to try to avoid patronizing children – children can feel insulted too and this can also serve to inhibit communication.

Respond to the child as an individual

It is folly to assume that all children are much the same. An over-awareness of stages of development can lead to the nurse lumping children into broad categories of ability. The only thing you can be sure about, when meeting a child for the first time, is that you are meeting a new person.

Believe the child

Trust forms the basis of any human relationship. Children's messages may sometimes appear inexplicable but flexible thinking and gentle questioning will often reveal the truth of the child's statements. Children must also have trust that the nurse is not going to repeat what they say to others without their consent. The child's right to confidentiality should be respected where this is possible.

Be aware of levels and stages of child development

While being careful not to categorize children too rigidly on the basis of this knowledge, an appreciation of this factor can help the nurse to pitch questions and response at an appropriate level. The child's response can be observed for signs of success in this.

Talk to the child 'normally'

It is important not to talk down to or patronize children. Some children resent the overuse of endearments such as 'dear' and 'love'. Every attempt should be made to keep speech clear avoiding complicated words and phrases. It is often helpful to keep sentences short. Communication can be rephrased or repeated as necessary based on the child's response. It may be necessary to break complicated messages into 'bite-sized' pieces appropriate to that child.

Think about the environment in which you talk to the child

Much can be done to help ensure the success of communication with children. A quiet, comfortable place with a minimum of distractions can help to improve the chances of the child concentrating on communicating and child and nurse fully understanding each other. This factor is particularly important when we consider how noisy places where children are can be!

Use play to communicate with children

Play is a natural feature of childhood, it is enjoyable and relaxing for children and as such can effectively be used as a conduit for communication with children. It is easy and natural to chat and play at the same time. This also has the advantage of being an alternative focus so that attention is not solely and intensely focused on the child. Some children find such undivided attention from an adult unsettling. Procedures which the child finds difficult to grasp can be demonstrated using a teddy bear or a doll. Play can take the form of modified role play to practise and rehearse new experiences.

Find out what the child likes to be called

Using the name the child wishes you to use is a basic token of respect. Equally offer the child your own name – introduce yourself!

Allow the child to determine how close you come

Children also require their personal space to be respected. Give the child time to inspect you and approach at a pace which is obviously comfortable to the child. A little thought will reveal that rapidly approaching and touching the child may be very threatening for that child.

Do not assume that the child wants to talk to you

It is an unfortunate feature of our society that children are usually taught early in life to be wary of strangers. Campaigns such as 'Stranger Danger' teach children that strangers can pose a threat to them. There is no reason that the child should accept that the nurse is automatically exempt from this. A gentle approach while the child can see that his/her parents accept the nurse is likely to bypass this difficulty.

The tired or anxious child may have a limited capacity for communication

The child who is afraid or anxious or tired may have a shortened attention span or a lowered frustration threshold and simply be unable to concentrate for very long on communicating. Again, carefully observing the child's responses and reactions can be helpful in determining the child's readiness to talk with the nurse.

Communicating with children in problem situations

Nurses often have great difficulty in talking to our children about 'awkward' topics such as the taboos of death and sex. Our society has intricate rules which govern how adults approach these subjects and children are often blissfully unaware of these rules. These subjects have great potential for raising strong emotions and the nurse confronted with a child who wishes to talk about such a topic may be very afraid of the child becoming upset. Again, before becoming embroiled in such a situation it is important to establish what the child, in fact, understands about any sensitive subject. The small child who blithely chats about death may not understand that death is universal (it comes to us all) and irreversible (once you are dead you do not simply 'wake up' later) (Dyregrov, 1991). To misunderstand this may mean that the nurse and the child simply remain on different wavelengths; at worst, the child may be frightened by the nurse's evident hesitancy and distress.

It is an old axiom when dealing with someone who poses an awkward question about an unpalatable subject that their motivation for posing that question must be exposed before attempting an answer. The questioner may wish to know exactly what is happening or about to happen and may equally well wish for a reassuring answer rather than the unvarnished truth. Time is necessary to sort out exactly what the child is thinking about and this time is also valuable because it allows the nurse to consider more carefully the response she is going to make and helps avoid the spur-of-the-moment blurted-out, ill-advised response. In this sort of situation the dependence of the child on parents and family is also apparent since the child's parents may have very clear views about what they feel the child should know about sensitive topics. For example, the parents of seriously ill children may wish to avoid the topic of death altogether. This is understandable since the matter is so painful to consider and they may feel that by avoiding the issue they are protecting the child from emotional pain and distress. This sort of situation requires a very gentle and careful approach. The child is often already quite aware that something serious is happening and may be frightened and anxious about unspoken horrors. The child may, in turn, feel that he is protecting his parents by not raising the matter with them but may be tempted to test the water by asking a nurse. There is obviously no easy way of solving such a situation but talking with the parents may clarify their views and motivations while suggesting means of approaching the topics of serious illness and death gradually and gently may allow the parents to be truthful with the child (Hill, 1994).

Ethical issues

When working with children, ethical issues are often raised and can be particularly thorny. Attention to some of the suggestions made above about communicating with children can help to establish an atmosphere of respect which can make a good basis for an ethically acceptable approach. A central issue is that of competence, the ability of the child to understand and make decisions about complicated situations, and this is often difficult to establish.

When considering the ethics of a situation the primary motivations of beneficence, or doing good, and non-maleficence, or avoiding harm, provide an orientation but often not a definitive answer. When talking to children truth-telling is, as with adults, the ethically acceptable rule but what is to be done if the truth might pose a risk of doing the child harm? One approach might be to establish what everyone in the situation knows or suspects and what the wishes of each of the key persons involved are. This information gathering provides a frame of reference from which the *rights* and *duties* of everyone concerned can be defined. When this is done the situation can be further illuminated by considering the potential *consequences* of each of the potential courses of action identified as possible. Such an orderly and rational approach, while time consuming, will allow properly informed decision-making.

Competence to make decisions based on a proper consideration of the ramifications of such decisions is a skill that adults are sometimes reluctant to allow the child. Of course, the very young child will simply not be competent in this context but older children are often surprisingly capable of dealing even with complicated decisions. The nurse may encounter such questions when, for example, considering children's ability to participate in decisions regarding their own health care and consenting to nursing or medical procedures. Our understanding of such questions is only now being clarified by work such as that of Alderson (1993).

Confidentiality is a right nurses protect without question for adults who use our professional services; this is embodied in our professional ethical code (UKCC, 1992). However, in the case of the child this right is sometimes compromised by our impression of the child not being competent to make autonomous decisions about the information they wish to keep private. The child's dependence on her family to act on her behalf makes it difficult to justify keeping relevant information from them even if the child directly requests that this should be done. Again, in this situation the case is rarely absolute. By discussing with the child the advantages and disadvantages of sharing information can be identified. Who is told what and in what format can be jointly decided. Ultimately, it is wise not to be rushed into making rash promises about not transmitting information. Consider the following scenario:

> Angela is a 13 year old girl who comes to a children's surgical ward for investigations of lower abdominal pain. When the nurse helps Angela to undress for examination Angela tells her that she has had a vaginal discharge and is afraid that she may have a sexually transmitted disease but that she does not want her parents to know that the is sexually active.

The guidance provided by the Children Act (1989) and consideration of ethical principles would indicate that if Angela understands the implications of not discussing this matter with her parents her wishes should be respected. At the same time, however, it might be considered that Angela is in need of the protection and guidance of her parents since she is clearly at some risk since she is practising unsafe sex. The matter could become very complicated if the nurse promises not to divulge any information to Angela's parents. The situation might change radically if it becomes clear that Angela's pain is due to an ectopic pregnancy. She would require emergency surgery and as a legal minor her parents would be involved in the consent giving process before any operation. This scenario illustrates how convoluted human situations can become. The important issue is that nurses do not approach such scenarios in a cagey, suspicious way, wary of being caught out but rather adopt a common-sense approach based on getting the facts straight and carefully considering the options for action available before making a decision. Brykczynska (1989) offers a wider discussion of ethical issues in the nursing of children which the reader may find useful.

Adolescents

The definition of adolescence is difficult to pin down but is conventionally held to be the period between roughly 12 years of age until around 18. Adolescents present a special challenge for nurses with regard to purposeful and satisfying mutual understanding and communication. The special characteristics of the adolescent who occupies the transitional zone between childhood and adulthood must be considered carefully. The adolescent will usually possess the ability to understand and reason much like an adult but may have less life experience to guide decision-making. Also, the adolescent may also be rather more volatile and erratic emotionally than an adult and this should be taken into account. It should be clear that the adolescent has a great many tasks to achieve in establishing who he or she is as a person. This includes accommodating their body image and personality and striving for independence from the family unit. These are arduous tasks and occupy the attention and energies of the youngster. As with children in general, an understanding of the characteristics of adolescence will help the nurse in communicating with this special group of people (Taylor and Muller, 1995).

Conclusion

Communicating with children in a purposeful way demands special insights and knowledge of the nurse. Counselling for children is a complex area, and the nurse should be aware of when referral to a specialist colleague, a child counsellor, is necessary. However, all communication with children has a counselling component particularly since, because of their special characteristics, communication with children often contains more of an information giving role than that with adults.

A careful, considered approach to talking to children in a logical and systematic way will help to ensure that this communication is helpful and satisfying for both the nurse and the child and family.

5

Counselling Nurses

Colin D. Somerville

Theoretical issues

This chapter is about counselling nurses. More particularly though this chapter is about counselling people. Nurses like all of us may have been hurt, battered, bruised and damaged by the experience of life. Nurses, who strive so hard to be professional, efficient, competent practitioners, can also be 'cracked vessels'. Nevertheless, things can always be different. Healing can take place even for those who, like nurses, so often have been taught not to show their feelings and to always be in control of themselves or, at the very least, to appear to be in control.

For over 11 years I worked as a counsellor with nurses. I had a nursing background myself so I was able to identify with and understand readily the pressures and practical demands placed upon nurses in their professional lives. Whenever I was asked, at a dinner party for example, what I did for a living, my reply, that I counselled nurses, always and without exception brought a response which referred to the demanding work that nurses do. Perhaps I should have expected this but I never failed to be irritated by this response just the same. I so much wanted my clients to be seen for who they were and not for what they did.

Asking for help, and even more, admitting mistakes or failures can be difficult for lots of us. For many nurses it is doubly difficult. Nurses look after others. So often the nursing culture does not give nurses permission to ask for help themselves, to admit mistakes or to take time to care for themselves. Besides, guilt comes easily to the nurse who goes against this culture. She or he so often feels that a nurse ought to be able to cope.

So ingrained is this that one of my clients laughingly used a phrase which has always stayed with me, she spoke of 'the hardening of the oughteries'! But nurses have private lives too. Nurses have mothers and fathers, boyfriends and girlfriends, and lovers and husbands and wives, and sons and daughters. Their relationships, losses and disappointments are every bit as real and painful as those of their patients. That hurt needs to be addressed, to be accepted and worked through and this needs time, patience and encouragement.

Ours is a society which is not too strong on encouragement. We are taught to be competitive rather than co-operative: to be concerned about personal success rather than the common good. In nursing, this is reflected in traditional nurse training and in the hierarchical structure of the profession in general. Most of us have been pretty discouraged in our lives one way or another and this discouragement we have carried with us into nursing where so often it has been repeatedly reinforced. It is difficult for us to see ourselves as being of value in ourselves for who we are rather than for what we do. We need time really to be listened to. We need to be valued and validated and encouraged not only as nurses but as people. For validation to take place some nurses have come for counselling.

My initial counselling training was based largely on the client-centred approach of Carl Rogers but over the past few years I have come to find that the principles of Alfred Adler's individual psychology are the mainstay of my counselling practice. Alfred Adler was, along with Carl Gustav Jung, contemporary with Sigmund Freud. In 1902 he was invited to join the discussion groups held by Freud which developed into the Vienna Psychoanalytical Society. Later Jung also joined the Psychoanalytical Society and Adler became its president in 1910. Nonetheless Adler was a colleague of Freud rather than a disciple. He had ideas of his own which were often in conflict with Freud's theories. Adler resigned from the Psychoanalytical Society, partly because of Freud's requirement for, ... uniformity and strict allegiance to his theory' (Dinkmeyer, Dinkmeyer and Sperry, 1987). After the break with Freud, Alfred Alder continued to develop his own school of thought and in 1912 his Society for Individual Psychology was born.

However the development of Adlerian
psychology has led to a significantly different
approach from that of the Freudian and
Jungian schools. Adler's point of principle, that
caused his disagreement with Freud and his
resignation from the Vienna Psychoanalytical
Society in 1911, was that sex or the libido was
not the fundamental drive determining human
behaviour. His view was that human beings are
always striving towards their own personal goals
– goals fundamentally decided upon in
childhood. Individual Psychology is so called to
underline the *indivisible* nature of the human
personality. Each human being is accepted as a
unity of mind, body and spirit and as a unique
individual.

(Adlerian Society of Great Britain)

For me Adlerian counselling and psychotherapy emphasize individual responsibility: the hope and possibility of change, the setting of realistic and achievable goals based on an understanding of childhood experiences and *mistaken notions*. Most of all I find the Alderian approach to be one of optimism and encouragement.

Adler gave great significance to early childhood events, birth order and *family constellation*. These are seen retrospectively in the light of the here and now. Our perception of the early experiences, which make up our own childhood's individual private logic of how to make sense of life, may frequently be based on misunderstanding or misinterpretation of events or circumstances. If, in counselling and psychotherapy these mistaken notions can be recognized then the client may decide to change his or her way of interacting socially.

Adler identified three life tasks. These are:

1. To express ourselves through work or occupation and so make our contribution to the community;
2. To find a way of co-operating with other people in society in friendship;
3. To find a partner with whom we can share our lives in the intimacy of sex and love.

Adler saw the three life tasks – work/employment, friendship/social life, love/intimacy – as embracing the whole spectrum of human existence.

> The human community sets three tasks for every
> individual. They are: work, which means
> contributing to the welfare of others, friendship,
> which embraces social relationships with
> comrades and relatives; and love, which is the
> most intimate union.
>
> (Rudolf Dreikurs)

The way in which we each deal with these three life tasks is demonstrated in the dynamics of our individual life styles. Co-operation and a concern for the welfare of our fellow human beings (and indeed for the whole of the created universe) is the way in which we best fulfil each of the three life tasks. Alfred Adler used the term Gemeinschaftsgefuhl, which is usually translated into English as 'social interest', to describe this concern for and involvement with the welfare of others – the common good – which he believed to be the natural way for human beings to live and to behave. However, because of perceived early discouragement and rejection, we often put aside co-operation for a spirit of competitiveness, self-centredness and self-interest. This leads to a life style which has little capacity for establishing satisfying personal and social relationships. This is a distorted life style. One that seeks opportunities for personal advantage at the expense of others and which leads to unhappiness and neurosis. Of such people Adler wrote,

> 'The meaning they ascribe to life is a private
> meaning: no one else benefits from their
> personal achievements. Their goal of success is
> in fact a goal of mere fictitious personal
> superiority, and their triumphs have meaning
> only to themselves.
>
> (Adler)

It must be said, however, that few human beings are successful in all three life tasks. For example, someone may be very successful in their work but less successful with intimate relationships. What is important is that, on balance, they gain their significance through co-operation with, rather than superiority over, other human beings.

All human beings are 'cracked vessels' but nevertheless we can move from a position of perceived inferiority to one of independent maturity and fulfilment. We can move from a life which seems meaningless and empty to one which is centred on 'contribution, interest in others and co-operation' (Adler, 1931).

How Adlerian counselling is used in practice

Elizabeth, a registered general nurse and a health visitor, suffered a major cerebral vascular accident when she was 28. She was considerably disabled and could walk only with great difficulty. Her physical disability had caused her to lose her role as a health visitor. This, together with general uncertainty about the future, was what brought her to see a counsellor. How could she come to terms with the losses she had experienced? Her loss of health. Her loss of the ability to function as an able-bodied person. Her loss of a sense of purpose and role in life. Her loss in no longer being able to function either as a nurse or a health visitor. Her loss of hope in the future and her need to find a new sense of belonging.

Adler's idea was that our primary need is to feel we belong. That we are acceptable, that we have our place and can contribute. People move towards self-selected goals which they feel will give them a place in the world, provide them with security and preserve their self-esteem. In other words we need to feel okay about ourselves. We need to feel we fit in. That we are acceptable and that we are valued, for who we are, as well as for what we do.

Nurses who come for counselling or psychotherapy, like other clients, come because in some way this basic need is not being realized. They are not experiencing life as satisfactory, in one way or another. Their sense of self-worth or purpose has taken a knock. They feel that they are unable to cope with difficulties in the way they have been used to doing in the present.

The counselling process

There are four stages in the Adlerian counselling process, they are:

- Establishing an empathic relationship between counsellor and client.
- Helping the client to explore his/her beliefs and feelings, motives and goals that determine his/her life style.
- Helping the client to develop insight into his/her mistaken goals and self-defeating behaviours.

- Reorientation – helping the client consider available alternatives to the problem, behaviour or situation and make a commitment to change.

(Dinkmeyer, Dinkmeyer and Sperry)

The client–counsellor relationship

The establishment of an empathic and trusting relationship between the client and the counsellor may not, at first, be easy. With some clients it may only be achieved after several sessions. It will require patience, openness and honesty on both sides. Nurses do not, on the whole, find it easy to admit feelings of inadequacy or distress to others. The Adlerian counsellor seeks to establish a relationship of equality with the client. The aim will be to make counselling and therapy a creative process which will be encouraging. This will enable the clients to experience sufficient safety in which to explore those areas of their lives which they are experiencing as unsatisfactory; to identify ways in which they may, if they so decide, bring about change. In some small number of cases the nurse client may feel that the mere fact that they have come to talk about the difficulties they are experiencing will be sufficient for them to begin to 'get things into proportion'. The new experience of having a counsellor giving them undivided attention for an hour, they may feel, gives them the chance to reassess their situation and see their way forward. Others however, like Elizabeth, will see the initial interview as setting the scene and/or may use it to test out the safety of the client/counsellor relationship. They may then decide to negotiate a contract of sessions in which to explore their difficulties in greater depth. The contract specifies the goals of the counselling process and the responsibilities that both the counsellor and client must undertake as equal partners in that process. The counsellor will give a brief outline of the way in which Adlerian counsellors work emphasizing the importance of encouragement and the possibility of change. This approach helps the client to recognize difficulties or problems as opportunities through which to learn and to grow and not as examples of inadequacy. The counsellor will also explain how confidentiality is to be kept within the counselling relationship. This latter point is crucial in establishing and maintaining a therapeutic counselling relationship. Every nurse knows that most hospitals have very efficient 'grapevines' and they will be anxious to be assured that information about their personal lives will be kept strictly confidential.

Exploring beliefs and feelings, motives and goals

> We shall not cease from exploration
> And the end of our exploring
> Will be to arrive where we started
> And to know the place for the first time
> (T. S. Elliot, *The Four Quartets*)

It is often the case that the presenting problem, although real, nonetheless is only a symptom of an underlying problem.

> Elizabeth was 30 by the time she came for counselling. She had a married sister six years older than herself called Margaret. Her father, William, who was a church elder, and her mother Beatrice were both 69. As children Elizabeth and her sister had their own secret name for their parents – it was 'the Mouldies'! Elizabeth described the relationship between her parents as one that was miserable and very destructive to themselves and everyone around them. Elizabeth said that she could see that there were elements of caring in her own relationship with her father, but, 'mostly he wanted to mould me into the kind of person he wanted me to be'. Elizabeth's relationship with her mother was 'very cold – she made me feel an utter nuisance and I never fulfilled her unrealistic expectations of me'. Elizabeth and Margaret offered each other mutual support in this household and they still enjoy each other's company. As children Elizabeth and Margaret experienced their parents as deprived, needy and overbearing people who attempted to mould their daughters for their own advantage.

Our beliefs, feelings, motives and goals are what go together to form what Adlerians call life style. Alfred Adler defined *life style* as, 'the wholeness of a person's individuality'. It is unique to each of us and is built on beliefs, perceptions and feelings about ourselves and others. Later in this chapter I will write more fully about a life style. The above passage, however, in itself gives some insight into Elizabeth's perceptions, beliefs and feelings about herself and other members of her family. It provides some insight into some of what goes to make up her life style. Non-verbal language is also very important for the counsellor in understanding the client's style of perceiving, acting and thinking. Adlerians believe we create our own life style, unique to ourselves, by the time we are seven. It is formed by the way we see our position in the family (not just birth order but our perception of our psychological position too), how we compare ourselves with our siblings, our relationship with our parents and our experience of the 'atmosphere' in the family. All of this the counsellor will encourage the client to share.

Helping the client to develop insight into mistaken goals and self-defeating behaviour

As children we are excellent observers but not necessarily very good at interpreting what we observe. It is like being born into a play which is being performed around us. Somehow, by trial and error, we have to make sense of what's going on. We have to find our part in the play. We have to find where we are, where we fit in and how we belong. We each form our own *private logic* about this but because we are not necessarily good 'interpreters' we each almost certainly have got at least some *faulty logic*. By encouraging the client to describe family relationships and early memories the counsellor can begin to see how the client's basic beliefs and perceptions influence the way they live, the way they relate to those around them.

Here are a few of Elizabeth's early memories:

'I'm about four and a half and I need new shoes to go to school. Both 'Mouldies' take me to the shop shop. There is a red pair and a brown pair which both fit. The assistant asks me which I like best and I say the red ones and my mother says she prefers the red ones too. My father says that red is a stupid colour and I must have the brown ones or he won't buy any. So we buy the brown ones.'

'I am in the kitchen. I am about 10. My mother and sister are there and they start arguing. My mother tries to strangle my sister. My father appears just in time and separates them.'

'I am about five. It is Sunday morning. I'm going to Sunday School and a neighbour arrives to take me. My mother tells me to go to the toilet before Sunday School which I do but when I come out she tells me I haven't been to the toilet and I must go back. I start to say that I have been but she pushes me back into the loo. This happens about 10 times before the neighbour in a very embarrassed way. He says I must go with him then or he'll have to go without me. She lets me go but tells me I'm a liar.'

'My mother, father and I are going out on an infrequent visit to some relations. My father's driving, my mother sits in the front of the car and I'm in the back. My mother starts ridiculing my father for what he is wearing. He gets very angry and they start one of their usual pointless extremely unpleasant arguments as the car is going along. Eventually he gets so angry he stops the car in the middle of the road, gets out and starts walking home. My mother curses and sneers at him. Cars are pulling up behind us tooting their horns and we just sit there with no driver and my father on the pavement walking away. I'm in the back of the car feeling utterly trapped. I can't escape. They are polluting my atmosphere with their unpleasantness. Eventually my mother turns the car round and drives it home. My father walks home and there is another pitched battle. I feel embarrassed, wish I was not alive and trapped.'

What mistaken beliefs or faulty logic might be revealed in this counselling process?

Here are a few of Elizabeth's: 'I cannot stand up to other people'. 'To be acceptable I must always be nice', 'I don't really matter' and 'I'm a silent spectator in life'.

The sharing which takes place between the client and the counsellor helps the client to feel understood and accepted. Once clients feel understood and accepted they can begin to have the courage to confront their beliefs and behaviour and begin to change.

Reorientation and making changes

Encouragement promotes movement from a position of a felt minus to a position of a felt plus. Encouragement is central to Adlerian counselling. It enables a client to liberate and develop the potential within themselves. It is brought about through a genuine interest and concern; sincerity; a non-judgemental and accepting attitude; attentive listening; giving responsibility and giving choices or presenting alternatives. The counsellor hears the feelings, pinpoints the beliefs but does not reinforce them. Instead alternative beliefs, ideas, achievable tasks and goals are offered. For Elizabeth these centred on beginning to be able to rely on herself and her own judgements, valuing herself and her own ability to choose, being able to state clearly her own needs and not seeing herself any longer as a helpless victim.

Christopher and his life style

'Yesterday morning after two days off I went into town to shop before work. Wandering around town, I felt vaguely uneasy and unhappy, about returning to work. At about 12.30 pm, I went to a bar or cafe near the hospital and had a light lunch. Still I didn't know what was worrying me. At 1 pm, I went to the hospital to prepare for work. In uniform, I went to the ward for the handover. Because they had had a very busy morning the morning staff asked if we could give out the patients' lunches, so we went onto the ward. Several of the other staff were talking very brightly and I realized I didn't share that bright feeling at all. Once on the ward I knew instinctively that I had to get away so I went straight to the office where one of the ward sisters was doing some paperwork. I sat down and told her that I didn't think that I could face being at work and immediately burst into tears. I know it is not work that is getting to me, it is an overwhelming feeling of being miserable, of not liking myself or loving myself enough. I feel it has been brewing up for some time now. I've been holding it back "bottled up" until yesterday.'

Christopher was in his mid-thirties when he first came for counselling. He was an enrolled nurse but was training to become a staff nurse. He complained of feeling isolated socially. He was lonely and had no close or long-lasting personal relationships and he complained of never being able to sustain a relationship with a woman for more than a few months. He was the youngest of four children and had two sisters two and seven years older than himself and a brother 10 years his senior. He'd been brought up in a family where his mother was 'the hub of the family' and his father, an Anglican priest, was a disciplinary figure who was always busy with his own work. The family motto was 'Do your best and don't worry your father'. Christopher said that he wished he had a friend he could love and who could love him too. He wished he had a house of his own and a better paid job and more time for writing poetry.

Christopher freely told me about his background and family and from the information he gave in our first few sessions it was possible to begin to build up a picture of what life had seemed like for him as a child.

When asked about his earliest memories he was able to recall incidents that had occurred when he was very young and which had left him feeling apprehensive, confused, baffled and uncertain about himself and his role. 'My earliest memory', he said, 'was when I was about two or three yers old. I was standing at the top of the stairs in a neighbour's house, in the morning, in my dressing gown, looking down the stairs, thinking about going down for breakfast but not really wanting to because it was not my own house. I often feel apprehensive because I am not always sure I'm really where I belong. I tend to be shy and am careful not to offend or to put myself into the centre of the picture. When I was about five I remember I took a plastic watch to school and showed it to another boy who was bigger than me and he smashed it. I was astonished and amazed. Even today I really find it hard when people reject my contributions or respond in unexpected ways.'

In two other early memories Christopher described situations where he was left waiting by himself – waiting for his father and waiting for the removal van when the family was moving house. In both of these memories there was an air of hesitation, passive expectation or anticipation which he agreed seemed to relate to his present day difficulties with regard to taking the initiative in relationships. 'As a child', said Christopher, 'I often found myself having to wait for other people's decisions or having to pull up my roots and move on. So it was difficult to really feel I belonged anywhere or that my personal needs were ever considered. Consequently I often feel unsure of myself in relation to others. I am careful not to offend and find it difficult to believe that people really care or can be relied on. I am disappointed when my expectation of, and feeling for other people seems very different from theirs for me.' Christopher mentioned another incident that had happened recently. 'I had a good friend come and stay for a weekend. On the Saturday evening we enjoyed each other's company and our choice of two video films: mine was *The Name of the Rose* and hers was *Jumping Jack Flash*. On the Sunday morning I got the Sunday papers and we had a late and lazy breakfast reading them. I then retreated into the kitchen to prepare a roast dinner which we ate and which my friend, Eleanor, appreciated. Then she resumed reading the papers. It seemed to me that she was choosing that, so instead of suggesting a walk by the canal, I picked out one of my favourite videos *Annie Hall* and began to watch it. Eleanor, having seen it many times, began sarcastically anticipating the dialogue, and when I protested that she was spoiling my enjoyment of it, she exploded angrily. She said whenever she visited me the first night was always very pleasant but by the Sunday morning I had got bored with her, and buried myself in my routine of Sunday papers and ignored her. She said that I didn't seem interested in her conversation and wouldn't make small talk, and if that was how I treated women friends it wasn't surprising that my relationships didn't last.'

Christopher has qualified as a staff nurse and now owns his own house. He has a responsible and well paid job but he still has difficulty with relationships. In counselling, his goals have been to learn to initiate contacts, to take risks, to accept and value himself as he is and to take on new responsibilities. He has achieved many of these goals already. He says that intimacy scares him still but he is able to relate to negative messages about sex and a lack of closeness within his childhood family relationships and particularly between himself and his father. With this insight he continues to work to overcome the mistaken notions which he established for himself as a child and which still get reflected in his present day relationships.

Problems and pitfalls in counselling nurses

'What you need young woman is a jolly good counselling! You have too high an opinion of yourself by far.'

Problems and pitfalls in counselling nurses fall into two categories – professional and personal. On the professional level the following questions are relevant. What is counselling and how does it differ from giving advice and guidance? What does counselling involve and what are the implications?

In many places where nurses are employed in the United Kingdom the word 'counselling' appears as the first course of action to be taken in relation to the disciplinary procedure! Is this appropriate? Not if we are talking about counselling as a therapeutic process freely entered upon between a counsellor and client. Is it possible to be sent for that sort of counselling? Many professional counsellors would think not. The British Association for Counselling has for long been concerned about the use of the word 'counselling' in relation to disciplinary procedures but the practice still continues. In particular it continues in relation to nurses. This fact alone creates problems and difficulties for those offering counselling services to nurses and to nurses seeking counselling.

When the dilemma arises between the use of the word counselling, where advice or guidance would be more appropriate, is presented to nurse managers, employers and the offers of a union or a professional body, it is unlikely to be challenged. In practice however, within the nursing profession, counselling will be seen almost exclusively in relation to the nurse's professional role. What the nurse manager wants is to help the nurse to be a better nurse and this frequently is only a very small part of what may need to be addressed in counselling. Counsellors would hope to help their clients to live, in all areas of their lives – work, friendship and social life, love and intimacy – in a more satisfying and fulfilled way. Counsellors will see their nurse clients first and foremost as people. Sometimes this may conflict with clients' professional roles as nurses.

It is not only the nursing profession which uses or misuses the word counselling in this way. The police counsel these days, so do insurance brokers, bank and building society managers, and double glazing salesmen, not to mention those working in the area of financial investments, careers, employment, housing and social work. Last, but not least, nurses themselves, without any specific counselling training, often present themselves as counsellors to their patients. What we should be talking about here is advice, guidance or the use of counselling skills, but that distinction is rarely understood.

The professional expectation, although not often verbalized, is that nurses ought to be able to cope with all the situations which they might encounter in the course of their duties. The implication of failure in this respect is that one is not suitable to be a nurse. This of course is poppycock. It will be strongly denied. However it prevails all to frequently. Few managers I suspect can honestly say that they haven't thought along these lines at some stage when confronted with a nurse who doesn't conform, has made mistakes or in some ways is considered to fall short. The nurse who is considered to need, or who asks for, counselling may well be placed in this 'not suitable' category.

On the personal level we come up against 'the hardening of the oughteries' too. Nurses are trained to be carers. They often feel they ought to be able to cope, be in charge, be efficient, capable, responsible, unflappable. Nurses ought not to panic. Therefore it is difficult to admit to insecurity, indecision and mistakes. These things equal professional failure. What will managers, colleagues, the doctors and the students think? Should I be doing this job? Am I a fraud? Am I a danger to patients or other nurses? All of these thoughts and questions may go through the mind of nurses under stress. It makes no difference if the stress directly arises from their work situation or from their domestic situation. Nurses are expected to take control in stress situations, therefore to feel under stress themselves can be hard to admit to. It is difficult, as was stated at the beginning of this chapter, for nurses to acknowledge that they feel inadequate, scared or unsure of themselves in professional situations. Frequently those who do come for counselling have spent many hours agonizing with guilt feelings in this respect. But 'we are all 'cracked vessels'. There will be situations for all of us, at some time or another when we can benefit from sharing our concerns, problems and difficulties. Nurses who can have the courage to admit this may benefit from counselling.

6

Counselling in Psychiatric Nursing

Mary Chambers

Introduction

The purpose of this chapter is to explore and discuss issues relating to counselling in psychiatric nursing. The chapter will focus on the nature of psychiatric nursing, the concept of counselling and outline how an eclectic approach to counselling can be used in psychiatric nursing. Problems relating to counselling in psychiatric nursing will also be addressed.

Counselling in psychiatric nursing: theoretical issues

Why, some might ask is there a chapter in this book which looks at counselling in psychiatric nursing when both are synonymous? Both concepts do appear to generate confusion not least amongst psychiatric nurses themselves. In a study by Chambers (1994) psychiatric nurses ($n = 39$; 13 students and 26 qualified nurses) were asked to describe their work. Counselling as a nursing activity was not referred to. However, elements of the counselling process were, for example, listening, creating a relationship, trust and support. For the purpose of clarification both psychiatric nursing and counselling will be defined within this chapter.

The nature of psychiatric nursing

In psychiatric nursing, unlike other forms of nursing, the nurse's presence is the main therapeutic tool. The nurse acts as a catalyst of change in facilitating patient recovery. This is achieved through a variety of stages of relationship building and through the therapeutic use of self. The therapeutic relationship and interactional processes therefore become the key therapeutic tool/agent in psychiatric nursing.

Interactional processes may range from being present and being with the patient and the use of silence, through to direct clinical interventions such as exposure 'in vitro' (Marks, 1987). In each encounter the nurse's therapeutic presence is the key to the healing process. The nurse is continually listening, reflecting, offering feedback and assessing what is taking place in the here and now interaction. Following each therapeutic interaction a judgement is then formed by the nurse in partnership with the patient. A decision is made about how to plan therapeutic care as well as the nature of the therapeutic modality. Being present for the patient is, for both nurse and patient, a dynamic process and one which carries a degree of vulnerbility. In other areas of nursing, the degree of vulnerability is reduced largely by carrying out procedures and/or tasks.

Psychiatric nursing, by its nature, is much less dependent on tasks. However, Chambers (1994) found that many of the interactions which qualified psychiatric nurses had with patients/clients were task-centred. Interactions that are task-centred reduce the vulnerability of the nurse, in that she/he is in a more powerful position than the patient/client by virtue of doing something to or for the patient (with his/her consent). In addition, the focus of the nurse–patient encounter may become the task and not the patient's feelings or emotional state. There will, however, be feelings surrounding the task in hand but, such feelings may be overt and therefore easily observed and not the covert ones at the heart of the patient's problems (Egan, 1994).

Definition of psychiatric nursing

Defining psychiatric nursing as a concept has been problematic for writers, researchers and practitioners. Many have referred to the lack of clarity with regard to the role of the psychiatric nurse (Reynolds and Cormack, 1982; Peplau, 1988). It was found by Chambers (1994) and Butterworth (1994) (see Department of Health) that practising psychiatric nurses had difficulty in defining the nature of their work. Chambers (1994) also found that the teachers of psychiatric nursing had a similar difficulty.

Within this chapter psychiatric nursing will be considered as an art and a science of positive humanistic activities which view individuals as existential, unique human beings. It is a process of building and developing a therapeutic relationship between nurse and patient. Through that therapeutic relationship and by using focused psychiatric nursing interventions, the nurse seeks to facilitate and maximize the growth, development and healing of the individual patient/client thereby enabling him to take an active role in everyday living. Embodied within this therapeutic relationship is a process of learning as both nurse and patient/client are on a journey of self-discovery. For the nurse self-discovery will be enhanced through reflecting upon the experience (interaction) and the meaning and significance of the therapeutic use of self.

Most of the literature available on the role and function of the psychiatric nurse emphasizes the importance of the nurse/patient relationship (Peplau, 1988; Reynolds and Cormack, 1990). However, much of the research material to date states that psychiatric nurses spend little time interacting with patients (Altschul, 1972; Clark, 1988; Handy, 1991; Chambers, 1994). A lack of planned structured time for therapeutic interactions results in a loss of healing time for patient recovery and therapeutic outcomes. More recently, Tyson *et al.* (1995) reporting on a small Australian study, indicated that nurse–patient interaction was higher than that previously reported, especially on long stay wards.

Counselling in psychiatric nursing

Counselling as a concept in nursing has often generated confusion. Not infrequently the term counselling has been used to cover a range of interactions from 'helping' interactions to 'being told off'. Disciplinary proceedings have also been couched within the language of counselling.

At the most simple of levels, counselling could be described as a conversation with a purpose. The purpose is to facilitate the individual through the process of self-discovery to maximize their strengths and achieve their potential. Nelson-Jones (1995) states that counselling can be viewed as a psychological process because the goals of counselling have a mind component in them and the underlying theories from which counselling goals and interventions are derived are psychological.

> In varying degrees all counselling approaches
> focus on altering how people feel, think and act
> so that they may live their lives more effectively.
> The process of counselling is not static, but
> involves movement of minds between
> counsellors and clients. In addition, much of
> the process of counselling transpires within
> clients' minds between sessions and when
> clients help themselves after counselling ends.
> (Nelson-Jones)

Regardless of how counselling is defined or described, the key ingredients are: relationship building, encompassing trust and mutual respect, together with a broad theoretical framework resulting in focused interventions to enable the patient/client achieve his/her goals. The similarity between the key elements of psychiatric nursing and those of counselling is immediately obvious.

Theoretical frameworks

Both Altschul (1972) and Clark (1988) suggested that psychiatric nurses by and large do not use any theoretical framework to guide their interactions with patients. Such interactions could therefore best be described as social and not necessarily therapeutic. This does not imply that they are not beneficial to patients/clients. Social interactions can provide a form of social intercourse which may well contribute to the patient's/client's sense of well-being and as such be beneficial. Indeed, there may be a time in the healing process when this form of interaction is more beneficial to the patient/client than highly focused therapy sessions.

Peplau (1986) considered such social interactions as one of the sub-roles of psychiatric nursing. She did not suggest that they had any form of therapeutic value. If all interactions were just social in nature or a means of gathering information to relay to medical staff (Powell, 1982), this would result in patients having reduced opportunity for self-discovery and healing.

Whether an interaction should be more social than therapeutic is something which the psychiatric nurse needs to be sensitive to and able to assess. This assessment will be influenced by the nature and depth of the therapeutic relationship which exists between nurse and patient/client. The assessment process will also involve an element of intuitive decision-making. Such intuitive processes are an integral part of psychiatric nursing as a therapeutic activity due to the continually changing dynamics of the therapeutic relationship.

Necessary conditions for counselling in psychiatric nursing

Regardless of the counselling model being used there are three separate but interrelated conditions which must be present for the success of a counselling relationship: person valuing, therapeutic ambience and the therapeutic relationship.

Person valuing

This is a necessary condition of all therapeutic psychiatric nursing and indeed all nursing. Nurses and patients/clients must *feel* valued and be *valued*. This sense of valuing has both an internal and external locus of control (Bandura, 1977).

The internal locus of control for the nurse is self belief. This means believing that what she/he is doing professionally is important, worthwhile and humane (Maslow, 1987). This contributes to the facilitation of good mental health. External locus of control comes from believing that what she/he is doing is valued by others in the organization, as well as the patients/clients.

From the point of view of the patients/clients the internal locus of control is believing in themselves. Some patients with mental health problems find this very difficult. Patients' self-concept and self-esteem are frequently vulnerable, damaged or fragile. Repairing and enhancing self-concept often forms part of the therapeutic process.

Externally for the patient/client, this sense of valuing is demonstrated by the nurse 'making time' to be with him/her and the giving of 'free attention'. Also, external valuing by the organization and the health care facility can be indicated through its care philosophy. It must be clearly demonstrated that the organization has the interests and health needs of the individual at the heart of its existence.

Giving of free attention

From the nurse's point of view the time which she/he spends with the patient/client should be uninterrupted, free from both internal and external distractions. Internal distractions may take the form of personal anxiety resulting from something which the patient/client might say arousing unresolved conflict within the nurse. Performance anxiety may be present due to lack of experience and not knowing how to respond to the patient/client. Wanting to get on well and be liked by the patient/client may generate acceptance anxiety. This may interfere or restrict the interventions used. For example, the nurse may not wish to probe or 'confront' the patient/client for fear of upsetting or offending him/her. This in turn may interfere with the nurse being accepted by the patient/client.

External distractions result from the competing demands of having to be somewhere else, for example, attending a case conference. In a community setting, the anxiety of knowing that there are a number of other patients to be seen on that particular day, spanning a wide geographical distance will create anxiety. The nurse, whilst thinking about these other issues, cannot therefore give 'undivided attention' to the present patient/client.

Therapeutic ambience

A fundamental component of psychiatric nursing is the creation of a therapeutic ambience. Therapeutic ambience is where the nurse conveys to the client her/his humanness and 'ordinariness' as reflected in both verbal and non-verbal behaviour. The nurse behaves as a real person who is genuine, free from pretence and superiority. The patient/client can 'sense' that the nurse appreciates and values his/her importance as a human being and accepts their totality as a person.

All interactions between nurse and patient/client are grounded in warmth and openness. The nurse sets aside all presumption, is flexible and responsive to the patient and not restricted by personal anxiety and rigidity (Heron, 1991).

By being open, warm, sincere and *ordinary*, the nurse becomes an almost transparent ingredient of congruence. Rogers (1993) considered congruence to be a key element of the therapeutic relationship. By relating person to person, one human being to another, in an open, honest flexible, supportive, transparent manner, the climate is set for therapeutic nursing. Creating this therapeutic ambience enables the patient/client to engage in openness with him/herself, which, in turn leads to insights and healing (Hough, 1994).

The therapeutic relationship

The therapeutic relationship is an integral part of all counselling regardless of the model being adopted. Such a relationship centres around acceptance, trust, respect, empathy, congruence, genuineness, warmth and unconditional positive regard (Rogers, 1993). Rogers has also suggested the importance of the counsellor being in touch with her/his own feelings in order to identify and monitor them. Heron (1991) emphasized the importance of the counsellor being 'present' for the patient/client and of 'giving free attention'.

Being present can be described as staying awake during the therapeutic encounter. Heron (1991) encapsulates being present in the terms of be *here now* and be *there now*. To be here now has been described by Heron (1991) as:

> You are centred, present, with your awareness unencumbered, in the moment that is now. It is nothing to do with your talk or social behaviour, but is all to do with how you are being. You are not distracted by concerns to do with the present or the future.

To be there now is an incumbent of to be here now.

> To be Here Now is very much also to be There
> Now. When you are attuned to your own centre,
> you are already very open to the reality of the
> other. Within the I is found the 'Thou'.
>
> (Heron)

The result of being here now and being there now is having free attention. 'You have active and directed presence' (Heron, 1991). This, Heron (1991) believes:

> Is a subtle and intense activity of consciousness,
> mediated by gaze, posture, facial expression,
> sometimes touch. It has the qualities of being
> supportive of the essential being and worth of
> clients independent of anything they say or do.
>
> (Heron)

Free attention is tantamount to being supportive and forms an integral part of the therapeutic relationship and therapeutic ambience.

Counselling approaches

No one approach to counselling is suitable for all patients/clients. Much depends on the nature of the problems being experienced by the person. The underlying principle should be that each individual patient/client is first and foremost a human being with their own special strengths and weaknesses.

Psychiatric nurses must be sensitive and responsive to the individual needs of patients/clients and not allow a particular theoretical approach to cloud their judgement or stifle their creativity. It is important that the theory or model does not become more important than the person seeking help. Today, in nursing, there is a strong emphasis on using theories and models of different types, for example, curriculum models, nursing models and models of counselling. These models, whilst helpful, can also be restrictive especially for the inexperienced nurse. They can create a degree of dependency and restrict the growth and development of the individual psychiatric nurse as well as patient/clients. Models and theories of counselling should be used as a guide, therefore manoeuvrable. They should not be considered 'tablets of stone', hence unmovable.

Nelson-Jones (1995) believes that one of the functions of a theory is that it meets insecure counsellors' needs for certainty. This provides counsellors with confidence which gets transmitted to clients. Others are much more sceptical of this form of austerity, for example, Hubble and O'Hanlon (1992). They see this kind of counsellor rigidity as counter-productive and describe it as 'delusions of certainty' and 'hardening of the categories'.

Equally important, the nurse should not adapt a 'cook-book approach' to patients/clients. This position is also more likely to happen with the inexperienced nurse practitioner. Lack of knowledge and/or skill will be demonstrated by the nurse using the same interventions and approaches with all patients/clients regardless of their appropriateness. In order to prevent this happening a system of supportive clinical supervision needs to be in place (Chambers and Long, 1995).

There would appear to be at least 16 different theoretical approaches to counselling as outlined by Nelson-Jones (1995). Some approaches are more generic than others, for example, the client-centred approach (Rogers, 1991).

In essence all counselling is client-centred. Behavioural counselling, for example, whilst adhering to a more structure, focused systematic regime is very much client-centred. In behavioural counselling the client sets the agenda for the treatment sessions and all goals are negotiated. The patient/client is very much in control of the therapy, therefore client-centred in the broadest of terms.

Levels of counselling interactions

Peplau (1962) talked of informal and depth counselling in psychiatric nursing. Informal counselling can best be described as that which nurses do in the process of carrying out a procedure. It has therapeutic value but at a surface level. There would appear to be a relationship between this form of counselling and the social sub-role of psychiatric nursing as described by Peplau (1988).

Studies looking at the role of the psychiatric nurse, for example, Cormack (1976 and 1983), Atlschul (1972) and Powell (1982) would suggest that much of the interaction between psychiatric nurses and patients/clients is at the surface level. This has implications for the role of the psychiatric nurse, as a skilled counsellor and for the education and preparation of future psychiatric nurses (Chambers, 1984).

Depth counselling appears to have much in common with specialist counselling and is a multi-skilled activity. Not every psychiatric nurse would be in a position to carry out such counselling. The current preparation of psychiatric nursing students is not sufficient to meet the demands of this role (Chambers, 1994; Watts, 1993). Those practising at this level will be nurses with a specialist nursing qualification, for example, a diploma in cognitive behavioural psychotherapy or community mental health nursing.

Another type of counselling is eclectic counselling where a wide range of therapeutic strategies are used within an integrated framework (Nelson-Jones, 1995). Using such an approach is also a highly skilled, multi-faceted activity requiring considerable skill and knowledge to move creatively between counselling strategies. This approach is more appropriate to the highly experienced, skilled psychiatric nurse.

Development of the counselling relationship

The counselling relationship with the patient/client usually begins with the nurse exploring surface issues. Patient/clients may have some reluctance about sharing personal information which is very private and covert and which may generate hurt as it is brought into the open. This is an understandable position, as no one would wish to disclose personal information to a stranger. Essentially, the nurse is a stranger until a number of encounters have taken place. Indeed the nurse may always remain a stranger. Movement depends on the level of trust which develops between the parties concerned.

As the relationship between nurse and patient deepens and trust develops the patient may disclose and confide more personal material. This results in issues being explored widely. At this point, the nurse may adopt an eclectic counselling strategy. As this relationship further develops, and the individual shares more of his/her difficulties, emotional pain and history of distress, the patient/client may indicate the wish to work on a particular problem. Here, the nurse may adopt a more focused approach drawing on a particular theoretical school of counselling, for example, cognitive behavioural psychotherapy (Beck, 1976).

The process of relationship development and the integration of counselling strategies will be dependent on the level of skill and knowledge of the individual nurse. The nurse can only take the patient as far as the nurse her/himself has gone personally and professionally.

This developmental process in terms of relationship building and the use of counselling approaches is similar to the three-stage map described by Cox (1978). Cox, however, conceptualizes the development of the client/counsellor relationship in terms of disclosure and cathartic release as outlined by Burnard (1994). Cathartic release may not always be necessary or appropriate for every patient/client. Much depends on the nature of the problem and the particular therapeutic approach being used. If the client is phobic of a particular object and the therapeutic approach is cognitive behavioural counselling (Beck, 1976), cathartic release may not be a necessary part of the therapy.

Counselling in psychiatric nursing practice

This section of the chapter will concentrate on the use of an eclectic approach to counselling in psychiatric nursing. Eclectic counselling is probably the most widely used as it is useful to a range of patients/clients. It is flexible and comprehensive and can draw from a range of other schools of counselling. It is also the approach that most experienced psychiatric nurses could and do use readily in their day-to-day work with patients/clients.

The example that follows is an excerpt from a counselling session with a young man, John, who was made redundant and whose marriage has irretrievably broken down. He has come for help as he feels let down. He also feels that he has let others down. He is holding himself responsible for the break up of his marriage. He feels unable to cope with an uncertain future, no job and little prospects of a job despite having a degree in engineering. At present he is in hospital and has had three counselling sessions with an experienced psychiatric nurse.

John knows that each day that nurse Jones is on duty he will spend between 30 and 40 minutes exploring and clarifying his difficulties. This is part of the agreement between John and nurse Jones. The counselling interventions which the nurse is using include catalytic, supportive, informative and cathartic interventions. Also demonstrated are examples of transference, counter-transference and self-disclosure. In this particular interaction there is no apparent structure. It is up to the patient/client to talk about whatever he wants to. Following an initial open question, the nurse allows the patient to take the lead.

After exchanging social greetings, nurse Jones asks John:

Nurse Jones: How are you feeling today John?

John: [Pause] Just the same, no change. Why were you expecting me to be different?

Nurse Jones: You sound as though you are feeling angry today John.

John: [Another pause] Look nurse, I know you are trying your best but is there any point really? You can't help me, I've nothing left, no job, no marriage, no nothing. What can you or anybody do? It's a waste of time.

Nurse Jones: What's a waste of time John?

John: You sitting there trying your therapy on me. Go and help somebody who is worth it, I've told you before that you're wasting your time.

Nurse Jones: [John is sitting almost directly opposite the nurse, looking at the floor and moving around in his seat.] From what you've said to me so far I get the impression that you are feeling a bit different today. Am I right, you sound more angry today?

John: Angry, depressed, fed up, what does it matter, nobody cares anyway, do they?

Nurse Jones: Do you really believe that John?

John: [Another long pause] Why is it nurse every time I ask you a question you answer with another question? Do you have anything to say?

Nurse Jones: John, like I said at the beginning, I get the feeling that you are angry today?

John: What d'you think, what d'you care? I'm stuck in here no-body cares, nobody came to see me yesterday, nobody cares.

Nurse Jones: [John fidgets with his jacket, he keeps looking at the floor, only glancing at the nurse very briefly.] Does someone come to see you every day?

John: No, not every day, but I thought my mother would be here yesterday.

Nurse Jones: Why? – Was yesterday special?

John: There you go asking more questions, what do you think?

Nurse Jones: I don't know John, but it sounds as if yesterday was important to you and that your mother coming to visit you was also important yesterday'. As I've said already I get the impression that you are angry today with everyone including me [Nurse Jones is beginning to feel a little angry as the interaction is not going anywhere. She, too, is also beginning to feel helpless – transference may be occurring.] John could you say what it was about yesterday that was so important to you?

John: Well, there's something which I want, no need, to tell my mum. I had it all worked out, what I was going to say, how I was going to say it. I didn't sleep the night before, working it out. Then she didn't come, she used to care; now she don't care either. [Another long pause, John was still sitting with his head bent but he seemed to bend over more. He was looking and fiddling with the corner of his jacket. The nurse noticed that there were tears dripping from John's face. She moved closer to John, touched his hand briefly and paused before speaking.]

Nurse Jones: John I can see that you are upset. If you feel like crying just let it happen, it's OK. Having a cry could help you. I sometimes find that crying helps me when I am upset or angry.

John: [There is a pause, John has tears dripping from his face, he does not look at the nurse but continues to look at, and fidget with the corner of his jacket. The nurse remains seated close to him, but does not say anything. This period of silence gives John space to cry, he does not feel pressurized into talking, he is allowed to focus on his feelings uninterrupted. However, he is aware of the presence of the nurse and of the security and warmth of their therapeutic relationship. The nurse waits for John to speak.] You must think I'm very stupid sitting here crying like a child. I don't know what has come over me.

Nurse Jones: John can you tell me what you're feeling at this moment?

John: I am feeling miserable, hopeless really, good for nothing. I have let my mother down, she worked so hard to help me through university. She did overtime in the factory, she took on other work as well cleaning jobs and that sort of thing. I owe her such a lot. She did not want me to do engineering; she said I had a better future as a lawyer. She might have been right. Look where I am now. I should have listened to her. I was stupid and now I have messed it all up. No job, no wife, nothing really.

Nurse Jones: John would it help if you were able to tell your mother how you feel?

John: That was what I was wanting to talk to her about yesterday. I wanted to say I was sorry for what I had done, to tell her that I feel ashamed and that I am not the person she thought I was. I lost my job then totally disgraced her when my wife left me. She takes things like that very bad. It is very hard to face her.

Nurse Jones: Would it help if you were able to tell your mother now what you want to say to her? I can be your mother and you can say to me what you wanted to tell her yesterday. OK?

John: No, I can't do that, I don't want to do that, not now anyway. I don't think I could. I was in the mood yesterday not now. Anyway it's not the same saying it to you.

Nurse Jones: I appreciate what you're saying John, but often people find it helpful to do things this way. It makes it easier for when they say it to those who they believe they have hurt. Does that make sense to you?

John: Yes but not for me, I can't do it.

Nurse Jones: All right John, but if you change your mind we can talk later. Do you think you are letting me know that you are going to have a problem telling your mum how you feel?

John: Maybe, you don't know my mum, she's a very strong person, she's a strong character, she wasn't very happy with me when I didn't do as she said about university. She was very disappointed, let down and all that. Now I've done it again, only this time worse. It's not easy for her to come to visit me in this place.

Nurse Jones: Why is that John?

John: Well this place is for people who are not able to cope, failures really. My mother has no time for failures, she was always on to my dad about being useless and not having any drive in him. I think that's why she pushed me so hard and wanted me to do well. She didn't want me to be a failure and look what I've done, just that.

Nurse Jones: John, I still think it would be good if you could say to me what you want to say to your mum, you may well find that it helps you sort out your feelings.

John: Nurse, I don't think I can, I'm not ready for that yet. Maybe it was a good job she didn't come yesterday. Talking to you has made me realize that I have a lot of things to say to her. Sitting here talking to you has got me thinking about a lot. I would like to spend a bit of time on my own, I am feeling tired, I could sleep. Can I have a lie down?

Nurse Jones: Sure that's OK. Thanks for sharing some of your feelings with me. I hope you found our time together useful. See you in an hour or two.

The above interaction highlights how the nurse through the use of a range of interventions was able to encourage the patient to move further along the road of self-discovery. The patient moved from feeling angry to being more reconciled and exploratory. He was more open to reflection and was prepared to give consideration to the suggestion of rehearsing what he might say to his mother. According to Nelson-Jones (1995) most of the counselling transpires within the client's mind in-between sessions. For John he was left with much to think about which may give direction to his next counselling session.

Pitfalls and problems of counselling in psychiatric nursing

This section begins by exploring problems which might arise within the counselling relationship and concludes by examining problems of a more general nature with regard to counselling in psychiatric nursing.

Problems within the counselling relationship

A common problem within the actual counselling session is the tendency, especially for the inexperienced nurse, to 'jump in too quickly' and not give the patient/client time to get his/her thoughts together. Such behaviour on the part of the nurse may be a result of anxiety and the need to be doing something. This could interfere with the balance of power within the relationship. The nurse, having a more dominant position, could lead the patient down a 'blind alley' (Heron, 1991).

Another pitfall which may occur with the inexperienced practitioner is the desire to prevent the patient/client crying or shouting. A not uncommon phrase used by nurses in such a situation is 'Don't cry, everything will be all right'. Such statements are misleading and may create a false impression or sense of security for the patient. Additionally, such statements could interfere with the nature of the relationship between nurse and patient especially if things do not work out. In using such phrases the nurse may be seeking relief from her own anxiety rather than facilitating or enabling the patient/client to gain new insights.

In order to overcome such difficulties it is important for psychiatric nurses to have access to a system of supportive clinical supervision. A culture of supportive clinical supervision will provide the nurse with the opportunity to bring such issues into focus and develop strategies for enhancing her/his practice. Another common pitfall is the compulsion to take on too many patients/clients. This compulsion is more difficult to resist for nurses working within a hospital environment. Here nurses are confronted with greater numbers of patients needing immediate help. This position is exacerbated if there are insufficient numbers of qualified staff to meet patient/client needs.

There is sometimes a tendency for nurses to attempt working with patients who have highly complex problems. The expertise of the individual nurse practitioner may not be sufficient to facilitate the patient/client achieve his/her goals. Such a position can be very frustrating for both, and in the extreme, has the potential to be emotionally hazardous.

Difficulty in disengaging from a relationship can create many pitfalls for nurses, especially those in training. In such situations clinical supervision can be of the utmost importance and benefit. The nurse may feel afraid to 'let go' in case things 'don't work out' for the patient/client. Also, should the patient relapse, the nurse may feel responsible (Chambers, 1994).

Problems surrounding counselling in psychiatric nursing

At a more general level a number of problem exist with regard to counselling in psychiatric nursing. One of the most critical is the education and training of psychiatric nurses in the counselling process.

Education and training in the counselling process

At present the initial programme of preparation for psychiatric nurses does not provide a strong foundation for counselling. The theoretical and practical preparation within the current P2000 mental health branch programme could be strengthened (Watts, 1993). Additionally, there are insufficient numbers of appropriate role models within the clinical environments (Altschul, 1972; Clark, 1988; Chambers, 1994). This position creates difficulties for those students and qualified psychiatric nurses who are interested in being more active as counsellors.

The experienced psychiatric nurse counsellor is a master craftsperson (Goldberg, 1992) who is able to integrate a range of therapeutic approaches and interventions, in a sensitive caring manner, to enhance the well-being of patents/clients. In order to carry out this work effectively, ongoing education and training is necessary. Basic nursing preparation is insufficient. The opportunity for nurses to avail themselves of advanced education and supervised practice must be available (Long and Chambers 1993). The implementation of the PREP (1994) recommendations will be helpful in this respect.

The tension between 'human becoming' and quasi-scientific measurement

The nature and process of counselling within psychiatric nursing presents problems in terms of measuring outcomes. The key objective of psychiatric nursing is to facilitate the individual on a journey of self-discovery and hence, on the process of 'human becoming'. This is a highly existential process and therefore different for each person. Such a journey is based on a strong therapeutic relationship which is largely of a low visibility nature (Brown and Fowler, 1971). Relationships of this nature are not amenable to evaluative judgement using the currently highly valued objective outcome measures. This places psychiatric nurses at the forefront of the debate of what constitutes quality of care, care outcomes and value for money. Such a position gives psychiatric nurses the opportunity to demonstrate that their work is highly valuable and makes a real contribution to health care. It also presents a challenge to those who wish to measure in a meaningful way the contribution which psychiatric nurses make. The real work of psychiatric nurses is not easily reached by the quasi-scientific measures and statistical analysis currently in use in the NHS. In order to begin to examine the outcomes and contribution of psychiatric nurses to the healing process of those with mental health problems greater attention needs to be given to the contribution of heuristic research (Moustakas, 1990).

Supportive clinical supervision

A further problem is faced when introducing a system of supportive clinical supervision. Supervision has long been associated with the role of management and not that of personal growth and development. This position must change if nurses are to take on a more active counselling role (Chambers and Long, 1995).

Taking on a more active counselling role places the nurse in an emotionally vulnerable position. Enabling patients/clients to work through their distress may well awaken similar stresses in the nurse. It is important that psychiatric nurses have access to a supportive supervision network in order to deal with these and other problems. The supervisor's role is to help the nurse, own, disentangle and make sense of any disturbing reactions which come to the surface during counselling sessions (Hough, 1994).

Supportive clinical supervision is necessary for personal enhancement and advancement as well as professional development and clinical skills progression. It is one way of ensuring that both the needs of patients/clients and those of the nurses are facilitated and developed in tandem. It is the responsibility of all practising psychiatric nurses to ensure that they have access to such a system.

Summary

This chapter has considered the nature of counselling in psychiatric nursing. Some theoretical issues and counselling approaches including desired therapeutic skills have been examined. An example of a brief counselling session was illustrated. The chapter concluded by discussing problems and common pitfalls that psychiatric nurses can encounter in relation to counselling. Finally, issues concerning aspects of education and training were tentatively discussed.

7

Counselling in Forensic Nursing

Marie Toman

Introduction

This chapter aims to provide insight into forensic psychiatric nursing and mentally disordered offenders, highlighting issues encountered within practice and resultant counselling. Forensic psychiatric nursing is a sub-speciality of psychiatric nursing, concerned with the care of patients suffering from mental disorder and who, as a direct consequence of their mental illness, offend, are likely to offend, or are non-offending but considered difficult to manage.

People who have offended may have committed sexual offences, man-slaughter, violence or arson. Power from and duty to legal bodies, i.e. the law and Mental Health Act (1983) regarding safety issues, social and political forces, faith, fate and culture, further complicate the role of forensic nurses, causing a rocky path to exist between society's needs and the well-being of mentally disordered offenders.

In the face of these uncertainties forensic nurses must determine their commitment. Is it to the smooth running of society or the well-being of the mentally disordered offender? Some would argue that a balance must be achieved between the two. Further adding to these difficulties, care of the mentally disordered offender takes place in secure conditions ranging from high to medium security dependent upon the level of dangerousness to self and/or others.

Secure conditions may constitute (and are not in any specific order) a special hospital, prison, regional secure unit and district services.

Maternal care or mother love in infancy and early childhood is considered essential for development and mental health. Indeed, abused childhoods, ignorance, inability to care, lack of guidance and balanced control may result in serious and consistent emotional problems during developmental stages and subsequent adult life. All form backgrounds commonly found among mentally disordered offenders.

Early action through child psychiatry and family therapy is often scant or non-existent, with the added effect on self-concept, self-esteem and relationships in general. Mental illness may be an outcome and as a direct consequence of the illness, some individuals offend to find themselves stigmatized, criminalized and viewed by themselves and others as essentially 'bad'. Mentally disordered offenders may be considered as individuals who are more sinned against than sinning.

Histories of ill-treatment or ignorance by others are often to blame when a child creates such problems as confusion, acute demands for love and nuturance, no capacity to care, difficulty expressing emotion and distrust in developing relationships. In addition, caring and relationship building may be further complicated where patients resent being treated against their will and/or find themselves clinically but not legally ready for release.

Counselling theory

Developmental and additional stated problems can be provocative to all; nevertheless nurses must first develop a relationship as an essential first step in activating a rehabilitation programme. Within this process and in representing the patients' best interest, all nursing interventions must be in context and sensitively applied. Interpersonal skills and personal attributes have emerged as the single, most significant influence on care outcomes, with Peplau's (1952) interpersonal model of mental health nursing exerting a meaningful influence on nursing and in particular the practice of psychiatric nurses.

Carl Rogers, a psychotherapist and member of the humanistic psychology movement, developed a client-centred approach, aimed at helping individuals towards achieving autonomy in thought, action and deed (Rogers, 1951). This approach, in addition to offering dignity and respect, provides a philosophy and foundation upon which nursing practice is based and care delivered within our medium secure unit. Staff supervision is performed by a psychotherapist who employs a Freudian approach to therapy.

Freud was the father of psychotherapy and as a concept it has grown, splintering off into many groups, displaying a marked tendency towards disagreement amongst its practitioners. Psychotherapy is concerned with emotions and involves talking about, expressing and understanding them. Unconscious or repressed material which is believed to be too painful to acknowledge and the cause of neurosis and mental ill-health is gradually made conscious, facilitated by the therapist.

The therapist is generally required to undertake personal psychotherapy and this is perceived as the only way to learn the process. Expression of feelings are focused on past and present events associated with parents, family and significant others. Expression requires the therapist to listen, question, interpret as well as talk, in conjunction with receiving personal therapy and supervision. Psychotherapy is not about telling patients what to do, or what to think. Ventilation aims to promote patient self-awareness about their underlying motivation for what they say and do, with a view to understanding them, and possibly changing, or eventually accepting them. Realization of bad feelings and associated behaviours does not equal a bad person and is therefore particularly important and relevant to mentally disordered offenders who perceive themselves as essentially 'bad'.

Client-centred counselling involves a decrease in conditions of worth and an increase in unconditional self-regard. Reintegration of this process requires successful communication of unconditional positive regard and nursing awareness that their own internal frame of reference does not impinge on the process (Rogers, 1951; Cox, 1988). Empathic understanding requires the nurse to place themselves into the patient's internal frame of reference. Achievement is through reflection, summarizing content and where appropriate, highlighting emotionally charged words.

Structuring a session requires nurses to be themselves whilst keeping a check on non-verbal and verbal communication; this congruence serves to highlight an essential skill requirement.

Additionally, the 'range' and 'depth' of interaction and spontaneous or planned silences, all call for careful monitoring of the complete process. Adequate structuring is particularly important when working and achieving with mentally disordered offenders and 'must be seen over and against a history' of major offence (Cox, 1988). Promoting mental health is initially realized through free association achieved at patient speed. Free association involves non-censorship from the nurse, along with patient-directed conversation focused on feelings, thoughts, memories, ideas and their relationship. This can cover a range of emotions with some sessions amounting to a slow and painful process.

Six category intervention analysis (Heron, 1975), a method based on interpersonal skills, is used in conjunction with free association, ensuring and achieving the stated balance. Emphasis, however, is placed on facilitative interventions, i.e. catalytic (drawing patient out), supporting (encouraging, confirming) and cathartic (release of emotions) (Heron, 1975).

Clinical judgement, range and depth restrictions ensure the patient's current mental state and their defences are concurrent with repressed material. To do otherwise could be counterproductive, leading to exacerbation of symptoms and or patient resistance. The process of self-disclosure also provides landmarks of progression which would otherwise be missed (Rogers, 1951; Cox, 1988).

Determining disclosure levels could prove difficult despite knowing the patient well. Here the nurse must discern whether what might be perceived by him or her as a superficial level of disclosure is the same for the patient. A system for 'coding the affective and cognitive material' and rating the same during individual work, is offered through 'coding the therapeutic process' (Cox, 1988).

Once this has been achieved disclosure levels are classified into the following three groups (Cox, 1988).

- **Trivial:** This is described as a first-level disclosure and reflects every day light-hearted small talk with the absence of personal disclosure, e.g. 'Good morning – it's a grand day'.
- **Neutral-personal:** This is a second-level disclosure and as the heading suggests is neutral. Personal disclosure, e.g. 'I'm interested in films'.

- **Emotional-personal:** The third and final level of disclosure reflects intense emotions associated with love and hate, e.g. 'No matter how hard I tried, I didn't achieve their expectations'.

However, the second and third levels must be considered against 'what it meant for the patient', before determining the level. In addition, 'genuine' third-level disclosure from the patient will be indicated through accompanying observable non-verbal behaviour (Cox, 1988).

This structure offers a way of coding, recording and describing the interactive processes between the patient and therapist which might otherwise become a confusing maze, providing a common language for multi-professional communication. Objective observation and knowledge of cultural and social norms are essential requirements in ensuring important clinical clues are not missed. This is particularly so in forensic nursing, where clinical clues assist assessment, providing indicators of patient risk and dangerousness and in meeting the demands of individualized care.

Counselling approaches

Complex presentation of problems are often associated with mentally disordered offenders who find themselves 'cast loose in stormy seas'. Primary nursing, aside from known benefits, offers mentally disordered offenders 'an anchor' through stability, consistency and a 'different experience' through a key worker relationship. The assumption that giving patients what they have never had 'will make them all right', unfortunately, is not the reality. The clock cannot be turned back, or significant other replacements given, nor past experiential gaps be filled. Instead and as part of the therapeutic process a different experience is offered and provides a foundation upon which relationships can be built with boundaries and limits set within counselling sessions.

Complex problems require that forensic nurses have a sound knowledge base in a specialism that can be drawn upon to assist the counselling process. Particular expertise is required in such areas as arson, self-harming and sexual offending. However, the generation of a nursing specialism is hampered by a lack of courses that specifically address and are of sufficient depth to equip nurses with the expertise.

Indecisive, inconsistent and easily manipulated nursing staff demonstrate a lack of personal control that may filter through into the counselling process. This can lead to patients feeling unsafe with some becoming assaultive, while others are fearful of losing control. In addition, undeclared disharmony amongst controlling staff and patients has the potential to cause staff to divide, further adding to patient and staff distress, hindering care and treatment.

Personal review through clinical supervision is therefore fundamental to retain objectivity, seek out how, why and under what circumstances patients and staff impact upon one another and devise interpersonal strategies for management and care. Empowering patients within a controlled environment can be a difficult balancing act in maximizing patients' independence and minimizing their dependence. Some would argue that a conflict exists between caring and empowering patients, presenting role difficulties for forensic nurses. Empowering forensic nurses in their decision-making would contribute towards maximizing patient independence and reducing role conflict. Good communication, de-institutionalization and higher levels of patient well-being is a concept that forensic nurses must constantly strive towards and promote at every given opportunity. Patients' rights, religious, ethnic or gender differences, social and cultural needs, risk and dangerousness are areas requiring assessment and attention within the counselling process.

The illness and/or the index offence (the offence for which they have been detained) may cause families and significant others to cut themselves off from the patient. Where family are part, if not all of the current problem, patient resolution may not be fully realized without their approved involvement and commitment. Throughout the complex process the therapist's role is very much as an enabler and therefore cannot force family involvement or patient change.

This can create a dilemma for forensic nurses where patient progress and subsequent mental health is dependent on collaboration and evidence of change. Where a patient is constrained by the Mental Health Act (1983) and the law, evidence of change is required before a patient can progress through the system. In this instance, this is from a regional secure unit to less secure accommodation or the community. Knowing and gaining patient trust is further highlighted and essential to achieve awareness of and early diffusion of potential danger signs. Strong feelings may be evoked through knowledge of a patient, their illness and 'index offence' (the reason for detention), potentially hindering development of a therapeutic nurse–patient relationship. Sensing nurses' fear may for example have the undesirable effect of enhancing patient anger or fear, or provide sexual stimulation. Other patients may continually push until an angry response is achieved and before trust is gained. On these occasions only, is it considered appropriate to display anger.

Knowing yourself is crucial within the counselling process, requiring nurses to monitor their behaviour, thoughts and feelings, ensuring patient communication is not blocked and objectivity retained. Monitoring emotions requires checking ownership; are they your own, or through empathizing, those of the patient? Own emotions require 'taking out', examining, putting to one side and, if evoked for reasons other than empathizing, they require discussion with an elected supervisor. Acknowledgement and expression of our own feelings will likewise assist nurses in dealing with client emotions and in retaining caring qualities and continuity in care.

Long-standing change requires that conscious material be assimilated within the personality; disclosure alone will lead to cathartic release and not much else. By facilitating the patient's thoughts and feelings with past events, the nurse assists the patient in understanding and coming to terms with them.

Patient involvement wherever possible, given the constraints, in decisions relating to their care, rights and activities of daily living, will assist in constructing a joint realistic plan of care. Individual need and background history will reflect on the nursing approach and whether counselling is formally timetabled into a patient's daily programme and or happens spontaneously.

The setting for counselling can be varied and requires that patient privacy, dignity and safety are ensured, as well as the safety of the nurse. Patient need and the venue will reflect on whether the nurse sits nearer the door.

Patient doubt about their ability to keep you or themselves safe can cause tremendous distress; this supportive approach will demonstrate your ability to maintain safety. Attentive listening is of primary importance and may prove repetitious and boring. However during the process, discovery will be made that some of the repetition has gone, acknowledging that the patient has worked through an issue sufficiently well enough to leave it behind. Ventilation of 'bad' experiences have to occur and become part of the resolution, before patients can talk about 'good' things. Change can be insidious and therefore missed unless acknowledged through regular evaluation to determine 'where are we at present'?

Some patients will experience great difficulty in verbalizing how they feel and struggle to find the words, others will not have the vocabulary. Linking current difficulties with self-expression and to how they felt in past situations is an important learning process. For example when children, some patients witnessed violent rows between their parents. Here self-expression is encouraged even to the point of struggling to find the words, before the nurse attempts to describe how the patient might have felt. Learning the use of words will eventually replace the use of fists, fire or self-harming when angry or experiencing raised stress levels.

As guardians, nurses need to be a 'good parent', and never judge, abuse or seduce our patients; physical contact – for example a hug at times of patient distress – may serve only to confuse and or add fuel to a patient's fantasy world.

Fantasy arousal and distorted thinking are examples of common factors when counselling and assessing mentally disordered individuals in particular those who have sexually offended.

Controlling, dominating, putting down, and anger are factors that can be associated with sexual fantasy, in particular with myths that exist about women and can lead to difficulties when caring and counselling, especially for female patients and nurses. Nurse gender therefore requires careful consideration when working with and counselling patients, as well as whether the nurse should counsel alone. Patient choice in key worker gender is another issue for consideration, for instance when a female patient has been sexually abused by a male. Patients may get angry and show it; nevertheless by still being there for them, this demonstrates you care and contributes towards a 'different experience'. This is highlighted when, and as treatment progresses, some patients express gratitude that you cared sufficiently enough to stay with them.

Past experiences may lead mentally disordered offenders to perceive themselves to be essentially 'mad and bad', irrespective of whether a crime has been committed and therefore whilst treatment is appropriate this may still invoke a response of anger. Anger is a natural response and if expressed may be associated with guilt. Some patients do not have the vocabulary to verbalize their feelings and or perceive words as all powerful and dangerous, preferring instead to express anger through fists, self-harm or fire setting.

Controlling their own emotions and behaviour produces difficulties along with fear of re-offending for some patients, with others seeking release by turning on themselves through self-reproach and or self-harm. Boundary and limit setting, within the counselling process, creates a safety net and assurance that this can be achieved on their behalf and until learnt for themselves. Maintaining control, through setting behavioural limits and remaining firm, demonstrates your belief in a patient's capacity eventually to achieve things for themselves, whilst making them feel safe. However, assaultive behaviour may occur through limit setting, reinforcing the need for nurses to know their patients and continue to use their interpersonal skills.

Counselling examples

Example 1

Patient: Things were getting really bad at home, with my husband's drinking and violence, my children and I were in constant fear. I had to work to buy food, etc., often we had to go without because he'd use the money for drink. I had no choice about the job, I had to take what I could get and my boss was always critical of everything I did. I felt as if I was going from one battlefield to another.

Nurse: Things were really bad for yourself and your children, you were in constant fear, you often had to do without. Also you had no choice about the job and with a critical boss felt as if you were part of a constant battle.

Patient: Yes, that's right, I felt that I was constantly being put down and abused. My husband blamed me for his drinking, saying that I was no good as a wife and mother and at work my boss was loud, he swore a lot, had a bad temper and treated me like dirt. What made it even worse was that everyone within earshot at work could hear.

Nurse: You have been put down, abused and treated badly.

Patient: They all did, I became a bag of nerves and it made me realize that what they were saying was true, even though I'd tried very hard, they'd found me out. They were right to treat me this way, because you see I **am** no good. After all my mother gave me away, so I couldn't have been good.

Nurse: You feel that you are no good because your mother gave you away?

Patient: Yes, she couldn't have loved me, otherwise why would she give me away?

Nurse: You were born at a time when being an unmarried mother was very much frowned upon and people generally would have made life very difficult for your mother to have kept you. To give you up must have been a very painful thing to do and says more about her inability to cope and was not because you were unlovable.

Through reflection of content, empathy was shared by getting into and responding from the client's frame of reference and this is an important early stage in developing a relationship. Reflection of content was achieved by paraphrasing or restating what the patient was saying. Additionally support was offered by affirming that she was not unlovable.

The patient perceived herself as unworthy of love and affection because she had been given away as a baby. Belief will lead to reinforcing the reality and so setting the individual up to fail. Misunderstandings between parents and children can and do occur and this is an area that can be addressed once the patient has ventilated the bad things and come to terms with their own feelings, which will then become part of the resolution.

Example 2

Patient: Staff are just making a big fuss about nothing, telling me that I was angry and frightening others, when I was just making a point.

Nurse: What do you understand by the word angry?

Patient: Well, that you had a go at someone and they can't accuse me of that.

Nurse: How did you make your point?

Patient: I only threw some chairs around and tried to smash a window.

Nurse: What made you do that?

Patient: They wouldn't agree with what I was saying, which just goes to prove what I've said all along, that they don't like me.

Nurse: When people don't agree with what you're saying, this means that they don't like you?

Patient: That's right, otherwise they'd agree with you wouldn't they?

Nurse: Well there are times when I disagree with what you're saying and it hasn't stopped me from liking you.

Patient: I don't believe you, you're just saying that?

Nurse: When you were a child, what did you feel when you saw your parents involved in violent rows?

Patient: Well it wasn't nice was it?

Nurse: That's right it wasn't nice, try and describe to me what your feelings were at the time?

Patient: Well, you know.

When others don't agree with him this confirms his belief system, i.e. that people don't like him. The patient's belief system and aggressive outburst are a repeat of his parents' pattern. It was important to clarify his understanding of the word 'angry' as words in general can conjure up many different meanings and images to different people.

In attempting to integrate current events, i.e. his outburst, with the past, i.e. witnessing his parents' violence, and the effect that his current behaviour has on others, the patient was encouraged to verbalize how he felt. The patient would be given every opportunity to find the words for himself and before the nurse attempts to describe how he might have felt. Here integration is an essential part of learning to understand the effect he has on others.

Example 3

Patient: I bet you all get great pleasure in controlling me and making my life as difficult as you can, don't you?

Nurse: It seems that when people control you, you perceive this as being cruel, whereas it's actually part of caring for you.

Patient: If you care about me then let me have my parole*.

Nurse: I expect you are feeling pretty fed up with being in here all the time.

Patient: I just want to be able to go out when I want to and not have to wait for permission.

Nurse: The clinical team makes this decision and will do so, as soon as it's felt that you're ready to make that step.

*Parole is a term used to describe when a patient has permission to go outside of the secure unit either escorted by a member of staff or alone and usually for a fixed time limit.

The patient's feelings are acknowledged, even though the nurse was not able to grant her request. The patient is still very young emotionally and with explanation of rules/guidelines, will go some way towards demonstrating the nurse's belief in her capacity to achieve things and the nurse's ability to keep her safe.

Counselling difficulties

Therapeutic custody will inevitably have implications for the nurse–patient relationship with co-operation and motivation towards treatment proving difficult, if not impossible at times. This is further compounded by no time limit on treatment received, further contributing towards patient powerlessness and poor self-esteem. Where relevant, the duality of the forensic nurse's role is firstly to protect the public and secondly to treat.

Self-harming behaviour and maladaptive responses to coping with anxiety might enhance these difficulties; forensic nurses are then faced with the demands and dilemma of witnessing patient trauma while at the same time counselling patients. Forensic nurses may also feel powerlessness and experience negative feelings towards a patient and should be encouraged to verbalize this in a supportive and confidential way.

Patients may present different parts of their personality to different staff, especially when more than one professional is currently working with the patient. The outcome can lead to confusion over symptoms, patient manipulation creating staff divide and lack of role clarity. Regular professional meetings are therefore crucial to maintain clarity of role and purpose and to minimize the risk of confusion and manipulation.

In addition, the parts of a patient's personality will have contributed greatly towards his or her current difficulties or crime. Collaborative working towards integration of the parts is therefore viewed as essential in treating the whole person and their mental health. Transference can be insidious and manifest in a variety of ways, requiring the forensic nurse to be on guard at all times. An example of this is when a nurse achieves a rapport on a first attempt, while another has been unsuccessful with the same patient after several weeks, with the patient continuing to display an obvious dislike for that nurse. A lack of discussion and subsequent insight can create inter-professional jealousy, or feelings of inadequacy and 'special patients'.

Although the 'successful' nurse is in receipt of a positive transference, this doesn't necessarily enable or facilitate any major work because the nurse is not in touch with the 'person' who has the difficulties. The 'unsuccessful nurse' however, is ideally placed to do much work, by assisting the patient to work through who the nurse reminds the patient of and why. Team support and supervision is crucial to assist the nurse with the hostility and difficulties of working in the 'front line' where the rewards may be a long time coming.

'Special patients' will also emerge, which occurs when the nurse and patient share a common belief that only one specific nurse can now manage their care. Other team members also come to share this belief, contributing to future complexities in caring and bringing about patient change.

When psychotic transference occurs, for example, when a patient maintains certain hostile beliefs about a nurse, then this can become very problematic with the risk of physical harm to the nurse. Fortunately this is not a regular occurrence, but when it does happen the nurse may be required to move to another ward.

Patients may have been transferred from another hospital where individual work has already been undertaken. Here the

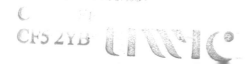

patient is well-practised at answering questions to the point of being well-rehearsed in their responses. This can make for difficulties in 'getting to know' the patient and 'real person' well, with all the implications for assessment of risk and dangerousness.

Keeping an open mind is necessary as a patient's view or memory of past events can be distorted with time. Intellectual understanding of problems is not sufficient; emotional understanding crucial to bringing about change takes a long time and will only be achieved at the patient's speed.

When neither the patient nor the nurse knows what to do next then it is desirable to acknowledge this and then add 'but let's keep working at it'. There will also be times when, having carefully weighed things up and made a decision, the decision proves wrong; this is a fact of life.

Nevertheless there will be times when we fail to treat and have to acknowledge and face our inadequacies, in particular concerning those patients considered seriously damaged. We cannot be omnipotent and this may result in a mourning process when letting go of the patient. Patients too will grieve and for all involved at these painful times and in addition to personal work, a suggested catharsis is through transferring thoughts and feelings onto paper.

Unreasonable expectations often continue after efforts to put patients in touch with the real world and it could be argued that such fantasies are what keep many patients going. Nevertheless patients have to learn to cope with their disappointments and realize that they cannot have everything that they want and this becomes part of their learning process.

Providing reassurance within the counselling process, for example as when a patient questions their ability to harm someone in the future, is very short-lived, as the patient's fear quickly returns and is therefore not useful as an intervention. Interventions that build on self-knowledge, coping and confidence are more likely to assist the patient in going forward.

Labelling people and its disadvantages are well-documented. However, awareness of the label attached to an index offence can play a major role in assisting the patient in coming to terms with the nature of their crime and the associated stigma in preparation for their eventual return to the community.

Conclusion

Forensic nursing practice has not been widely written about and yet presents the profession with unique and complex challenges which also have relevance to psychiatric nursing practice.

Society's view of the mentally disordered offender is generally unsympathetic and greatly influenced by media sensationalism. Forensic nurses will also find themselves stigmatized and working against current public opinion, and therefore need to possess principles that are not easily destroyed by criticism. Raising public awareness and conscience to the plight of mentally disordered offenders must be owned and actioned by all who care, and must become a priority if this immoral cycle is to be halted. This may only be achieved through increased information which will lead to destigmatizing a doubly stigmatized group.

Interpersonal skills play an essential role in facilitating patient change both within and outside formal counselling sessions. Self awareness and retaining a sense of self during patient and staff interactions are crucial to the provision of a therapeutic environment and the process of patient change. It is desirable therefore that forensic nurses employ these skills throughout an entire span of duty.

Gaining patient trust in addition to trusting the patient has been identified as essential within the therapeutic process. Additionally crucial is the maintenance of the patient, nurse and society's safety and this is achieved only through knowing the patient. Trusting that the patient will or will not do something remains open to subjective assessment and it may be that total objectivity cannot be achieved.

Nevertheless, identification and rigorous recording of core determinants within the decision-making process, can only provide a way forward to a more accurate measurement of risk and dangerousness. The extent to which nurse–patient relationships produce change and/or psychopharmacology influence patients' behaviour is open to debate, further demonstrating the need for reliable assessment tools wherever practicably possible. Cox's (1988) system for coding offers a solution and way forward. While it is fully appreciated that each client situation is unique and interventions can never be strictly copied, core problems do exist and are common to more than one patient.

All these pointers suggest an urgent need for forensic nurses, to provide evidence of their effectiveness. Difficulties encountered during the counselling process emerge as man-made and can be imposed by the wider management agenda and the law. The business management agenda for example is concerned with a constant drive to achieve 'value for money', 'efficiencies' and business planning outcomes. This can impact on care outcomes as perceived by patients, their relatives and carers. In accepting the legal and security constraints, management decisions need to be responsive to this impact. 'Bottom up' feedback is an identified and effective way to achieve desired quality standards and change existing policy which now forms the basis for service level agreements and contracts.

Empowering forensic nurses in making decisions directly concerned with care management, as well as being made accountable for these decisions, can only assist in furthering patient empowerment and raising their self-esteem.

Where more than one professional is involved in a patient's treatment programme and in further supporting the above suggested change, the forensic nurse would act as 'gatekeeper' and having firstly taken into consideration the patient's needs, would make certain these needs were met, further contributing to continuity of care.

Counselling theory and practice within forensic nursing demonstrates the necessary knowledge and skill required to be effective practitioners in meeting the complex problems associated with mentally disordered offenders. Clinical supervision would support and ensure that difficult management problems and negative feelings do not impact on patient care and retain physical and mental health of forensic nurses. Forensic nursing practice however remains ill-defined, requiring a sound knowledge base that will question, define and direct the profession achieving and promoting mental health.

8

Counselling in Crises

Bob Wright

Crisis is an inevitable part of the human experience. People are constantly confronted with situations which threaten their ability to function. Some of these situations cannot be resolved by customary methods and there is a need to seek professional assistance. For a time, customary methods may not offer enough resources to overcome the difficulty. Family and friends may also be experiencing some of the disorder produced by the event, or may be less readily available to help due to our mobile society.

Crisis intervention is a direct and active entering into the current life event in order to help the client mobilize resources and regain control.

Regardless of the nursing area in which they work, nurses are constantly facing clients who are in a potential state of crisis. Medicine, surgery, obstetrics and gynaecology, as well as the victims of road traffic accidents, are some of the areas of nursing care where clients can be in crisis. Whilst my area of crisis counselling is in the emergency department, the concepts apply to all areas of care.

Theoretical approaches

Eric Lindemann's contribution to the theory of crisis intervention is based on the Coconut Grove fire of 1944 and an acute reaction to grief (Lindemann, 1944). He concluded that this fire (in a night club) resulted in a crisis for all individuals closely involved, and that most went on to experience a normal grief reaction. The study highlights how counsellors do not take control of the individual but help him to move into normal coping processes.

This aspect of crisis theory, introduced by Lindemann, was described in more depth by Caplan (1964). In Caplan's theories about life crisis he acknowledged the influence of Erikson's model of developmental (maturational) and situational (accidental) crisis. Caplan described developmental crises as transitional periods in personality development, characterized by disturbances in affective and cognitive functioning. A sudden unexpected threat, or loss of basic resources or life goals, constitutes a situational crisis.

Situational crises, which form the majority of my work, are not as common as developmental crises and they result in more intense periods of psychological and behavioural disorganization. Caplan observed that as most of these situations are new to the clients, their usual coping methods did not work. Caplan concluded that there are universal responses to crisis. Even individuals with a relatively stable personality may change in unexpected ways during a crisis.

The change needed to deal with a crisis may have positive aspects which highlight the opportunities that crisis can bring. On the other hand the crisis can lead to an increased inability to cope, and to feelings of chaos and disorder. This notion leads to the view that a crisis is a transitional period that offers the individual an opportunity for growth or for greater vulnerability.

Time is another aspect to consider. A crisis, by its very nature, cannot last for a long period because it involves intensely difficult feelings of distress and disorder. We could not tolerate these feelings for very long as they have the capacity to damage. So time has implications for the crisis counsellor – the nature of the work means we have to move in quickly and offer frequent and lengthy periods of counselling at the impact of the crisis, in order to prevent damage and help restore some equilibrium.

Caplan viewed crisis intervention as a major part of preventative psychiatry. He believed that individuals could be supported and taught to deal more effectively with the crisis and so prevent mental disorders. This primary prevention is the promotion of mental health and offers the client a model with which to manage the disorder in all the dimensions of his person.

Most theorists accept Caplan's premise that a crisis situation is self-limiting, lasting from one to five weeks. The focus of the counselling is the client's current life experience relating to the crisis. The client's previous experiences, relating to unsolved conflict, are part of the counselling only as far as their influence on the current work.

Beginning to work with crisis

For most people, the sudden death or serious injury of someone close produces a period of disarray. This is seen on a cognitive, behavioural and feeling level, and adds to the whole experience of disorder or loss of control. To begin to manage the event is to put the incident in the present context, grasping some of the reality and introducing some order again. The three factors of Caplan's framework describe the areas of difficulty to be worked with.

1. Perception of the event	2. External resources	3. Inner resources

Figure 8.1 *Caplan's framework for working with crisis*

1. Perception of the event

The client's realistic appraisal of the event is important. Its impact and ability to produce disorder are very apparent at this stage. There may be painful expressions of what this event means to hopes, aspirations and plans. Questions will emerge, some repeatedly, highlighting a need to have a better perception of what is happening. This event does not fit into current plans; it is an awful imposition and a threat. Some people will need to protest and to reject information given to them.

2. External resources

External resources are the second factor to work with at the time of impact. Sometimes it is obvious that the client can readily identify and access external resources, but others are prevented from doing this by the cognitive disarray. Agitation, hyperactivity, and an inability to concentrate will all prevent the client from accessing people efficiently.

Most people know and say who they instinctively need. To access them is usually the problem. Some will need us to introduce them to external resources which will help them work with their crisis.

3. Inner resources

The client may find some inner resources or coping mechanism to help him manage his feelings. With many crises the problem is that we have no previous experience of this type of event from which to recall strategies. The fear produced can result in the client being immobilized, and this in turn can lead to panic measures. At the time of impact, it is very common for clients to deny having any inner resources.

The theory is that if we can help the client to look at and work positively with the three factors, a crisis may be averted. The three factors then are:

1. The client's perception of the event.
2. External resources.
3. Inner resources.

If denial of the meaning or the reality of the event is paramount, then the first factor has a strong negative content. If external resources are poor or not available, then the second factor has a strong negative content.

The individual's difficulty in locating resources or strengths or insights within himself will make the third factor a nonproductive exercise.

One or two negative responses to the three factors are likely to take the client into a life crisis.

To summarize so far

A crisis occurs when an individual is faced with an insurmountable obstacle which affects his life's aims and threatens his very existence. The usual methods of problem solving are ineffective, and he becomes disorganized. Intense efforts are made to solve the problem, and past anxieties may interfere with the individual's ability to organize himself. Intervention should deal with the immediate crisis and he will need your help to do this.

Before dealing with the crisis it will be ascertained that the individual concerned has no known classification of mental illness as far as is possible during an initial discussion.

Each phase below describes a level of the crisis. The four phrases of crisis are summarized in Figure 8.2 whilst Figure 8.3 (overleaf) describes the phrases in greater detail, thereby defining the focus for each phase.

Phase	*Intervention*
Phase 1	May be resolved by routine coping mechanisms
Phase 2	May be resolved by trying on a trial and error basis
Phase 3	May be resolved by redefining the situation or the motives of the individual, or both
Phase 4	Is a description of a severe state of crisis where an individual has insufficient resources to cope

Figure 8.2   *The four phases of crisis*

As the client moves towards Phase 3 his struggle will be obvious to the counsellor, as will his distress at finding nothing to help him make the crisis more manageable. He will become less responsive to the counsellor's efforts to help him, becoming easily distracted, often with trivia. His span of concentration will diminish and he may even be dismissive of the counsellor.

This shift towards devaluing the counsellor's role, his inability to stay with the focus and, his poor span of attention are all signs of an increasingly distressed and more difficult client. This occurs just before Phase 4 when, as Figure 8.3 shows, the client is in a severe state of crisis.

Phase	*Counselling focus*
Phase 1 A threat occurs which produces strain, tension. It attacks basic self-esteem needs.	May be resolved by routine coping mechanisms. Past experience may come up with an answer.

Failure to resolve leads to

Phase 2 Past experience offers little or nothing. Tension increases. Feels helpless and hopeless.	May be resolved by looking at alternatives. The patient may try different responses on a trial and error basis and choose the most acceptable.

Failure to resolve leads to

Phase 3 Intense activity. Disorder/disorganization. Old anxieties recur. Preoccupation with trivia. Make or break action.	May be resolved by redefining the focus. This brings the event down to a manageable size. Work with today. Helper takes on a more direct approach.

Failure to resolve leads to

Phase 4 Failure to resolve. Withdrawal. Hopelessness. No longer able to cope. No resources to handle it.	A severe state of crisis. Person needs comfort, a listening ear without judgements, a peaceful environment, respite from struggle to solve the problem.

Figure 8.3   *The four phases of crisis with counselling focus*

Crisis counselling

Firstly we should consider the word 'counselling', a word which is often used inappropriately. You will sometimes hear about a nurse being counselled when disciplinary measures are being taken. Although we will not be examining the nature of counselling in depth it must be stressed that it is totally removed from anything of a punitive nature.

As far as the nurse is concerned, the task of counselling involves exploring and examining the present situation with the client and/or his family. This is not an intellectual exercise but must involve the feelings of the client, and this is undertaken by helping him to feel safe with you, the counsellor.

The hospital, and you as its representative, may be perceived as a threat for many reasons. Being a uniform, for example, may cause some difficulty about your being recognized as an individual. You may be seen as someone who will defend and promote the institution (the hospital) above all else. Hopefully, your empathy and individuality will help you understand the client's difficulties and feelings.

Firstly, you have on offer your own humanity. In my view this comes before your role as a nurse. Your being a nurse may interfere with the transaction, and your concern for the pain, distress and difficulty needs to be communicated both verbally and physically. Many nurses deny or are diffident about the skills they have to offer. To deny any ability or skill is as unrealistic as feeling able to sort out any problem. A desire to see a rapid solution will cause you problems. In a busy ward or department, time can become an all important factor. When you believe in the real value of the intervention you will feel less threatened by the time factor.

Giving advice which the client is unable to carry out is to be avoided. It will increase your sense of inadequacy and is not useful. Your acceptance of the individual and what he or the family brings is of immense value. You do not have to agree with the lifestyle or morals or behaviour of the client or his family. You are responding to emotional anguish, pain and distress.

Because of strong personal feelings there may be occasions when someone else should be involved. This may occur if you have strong religious or ethical values which may be compromised. If you are unable to opt out of the situation, you will need to be aware that these values might interfere inappropriately with the transaction. This can be very difficult. Imagine having to treat a self-poisoned child rapist or murderer. The feelings produced can be so powerful as to be overwhelming. In this situation you come to appreciate the value of space ('time out') to discharge feelings and air views after the event.

It can be difficult to stick with the feelings especially if you are in a hurry. Due to the many demands on your time you may have to move the situation along faster than it would develop naturally. But if this is done along with the client, it may not be felt as a rejection. Since time is such a disturbing factor in crisis, such movement will often not be a problem, because movement feels much more comfortable than stasis.

The nurse can help the client and his family to say what they think and feel. This confrontation of feelings can lead to resolution of difficulties, because so often it is the unspoken that delays resolution. All nurses know about and have experienced this. You will recall the anger you have felt when you knew the diagnosis and prognosis of a patient and have been obliged to avoid the whole subject. Sharing and exploring the feelings associated with the crisis may give clients greater understanding of their particular response and behaviour, and will help remove their fear that the crisis is making them 'go mad'.

It would be a mistake to believe that you can solve the client's problems – only he can do that. However, you can be instrumental in beginning the process of coping with the crisis. You may set the pattern for a healthy supportive process which helps change to take place. Setting the pattern may involve helping the patient or his family to identify the factors which produced the crisis. Rosemary Johnson (1980) calls these the balancing factors. They are listed as the realistic perception of the event, the emotional supports and the coping mechanisms.

Exploring and clarifying the various aspects of these balancing factors can open the way to resolution.

My work in the UK and the work I have observed in the USA have been labelled in various ways (Wright, 1993). Some would call it 'crisis counselling', others 'crisis intervention'. Many would regard it as 'supportive therapy' or 'grief work'. You may stick rigidly to the crisis mode and intervene in Phase 2 and not see the crisis abating. But although you may not see any alteration yourself – because of the brevity of your intervention – you may set a pattern. This is the pattern which helps individuals to find the resources to cope.

Crisis counselling in practice

Victims of violence

An increasing number of our emergency patients are the victims of violence. For these victims, the injury with which they present is often felt to be less of a problem than the overall psychological implications of the event. This in itself can be a hazardous situation in our overall evaluation of the patient. For example, the person who is coshed and robbed of a large amount of money may trivialize a serious injury because of his feelings of violation and revenge. We must not overlook the injury.

Suffering at the hands of another person results in various responses. Victims may not only feel they will continue to suffer and be oppressed, but also that they are to blame. There is a strong sense of lack of control over their life and that some weakness or poor judgement on their part caused the event.

We see protest and also withdrawal and helplessness. Some victims appear unhelpful or just unresponsive, and the passivity can irritate those around them. The focus of difficulty shifts rapidly from the event to aspects of life important to the victim. Irrational though this may seem to others, the event permeates all that the victim values, and attacks his belief system and future prospects.

> Mrs Smith, aged 80 and widowed for 10 years, lived in a small house in a long terrace, in a run-down area of the city. She did not want to move although often encouraged to do so by her two married sons, both successful and living in more affluent areas of the city. She was happy here, with good friends and neighbours and happy memories of her husband and bringing up the children. It was familiar territory.
>
> On a Monday evening in February, she accompanied her friend Alice to the local social club. It was a dark, wet evening. Just before arriving at Alice's front door, only a few hundred yards from her own, she heard running footsteps behind her and being a happy, contented person, felt them to be no threat.
>
> Suddenly she was pushed and felt her handbag being dragged from her. She protested, surprised and affronted:

'What do you think you are doing?' hanging onto the bag at the same time.

'Let go you old cow' the youth shouted, and pulled her to the ground.

'Like hell you little bastard', she heard herself saying, whilst losing the fight to retain the bag. A searing pain shot through her arm and shoulder and she felt sick with pain and fear.

Before he finally took control of the bag he punched her hard in the face.

When she told me this story, Mrs Smith was lying on a trolley in the A and E department, undressed and in a white gown, covered with a blanket. The nurses told me how ashamed she was that she had been incontinent of urine and had asked them not to let anyone see her soiled underclothes. Her sons had been contacted but only one was available and he was on his way.

Perception of the event – Mrs Smith

'My son will be really angry with me. He is always saying I should move to a nicer area. I don't want to lose my home, my friends, my memories, my feeling of being near the happiest moments of my life. I won't be able to go out alone any more. That's terrible; I value my independence.

'It was my fault. I heard him approaching and did nothing about it. I should not carry all that money. You won't tell my son what I called the thief, will you? I cannot believe I could say that. You must think I am terrible. I just want to go home but how can I? I've made a complete mess of everything.'

Perception of the event – Mrs Smith's son

'She is stubborn. She will not listen. We do not want her to live there. She has been stupid going out alone and in the dark. What do you do? They won't listen. We have money. She has no need to live like that. Why is she being kept waiting? Do something now.

'Half these other patients are a waste of time, they deserve what they get. She can never return there. I have no option but to take her home to live with us. We really have not the room.

It will cause chaos at home. My wife goes out to work. I have no choice. She is my mother.'

The interaction between mother and son was tense and sad, both apologizing to each other, the son becoming angry and controlling. He had to make the decision for her. She would have to live with him. Mrs Smith became withdrawn, emotionally flat and apathetic: 'Do what you want, I don't care any more'.

The fracture was re-positioned and immobilized, and it was decided to admit her overnight to re-evaluate the injury the following morning and for better pain control. This also gave us an opportunity to offer crisis counselling, and using the three factors of crisis to introduce some feeling of regaining control again.

As described previously, on impact her perception of the event took up most of the time, and strong negative factors distorted the whole event. No external resources other than the sons were perceived. Inner resources offered very little. The nursing care should have established some good conditions in which to begin the further evaluation. In brief, this care for victims should establish the following:

1. **Confidentiality:** Sensitive and embarrassing aspects will not be disclosed and the patient's privacy will continue to be valued.
2. **Establish safety, and confirm reality:** Explain who you are, your role, and your offer of help. Touching, explaining, confirming what has happened.
3. **Help her to share feelings:** Ask what happened. Provide feedback so that she knows you hear and understand. This helps validate the feelings associated with the incident.
4. **Remove signs of damaged clothing, dirt, blood, etc:** Allowing the victim to shower, wash, removes feelings of contamination. Re-establish 'clean' state.
5. **Involve her in decisions made about her:** Removes feelings of helplessness and dependency.
6. **Deal with sense of isolation:** Do not leave alone for long periods.
7. **Remember not to reinforce blame or guilt:** It is easy for the nurse to do this.

Twelve hours later

Mrs Smith is sitting in our short stay ward, which has windows. It is now daylight, another day, something that should be remarked upon. Another chance to re-tell the story. Away from the chaos and disorder of the immediate impact, some details will be further clarified. Opportunity will arise to remind her of the stalwart, determined way she approaches life.

'It must have been difficult, bringing up children when times were harder.'

'You obviously did a good job.'

'It took that robber some effort to get that bag from you.'

'You are tougher than you think.'

'You sound as if you gain so much from living there.'

'We are talking about an incident which lasted three minutes in your 80 years.'

Without telling her how she feels, we are checking out any changes in her perception of the incident. Last night she saw impending loss of many aspects of her life which were important to her. Perhaps that strength and determination she exhibits will be an asset to her. Will this mean rediscovering the inner resources she needs?

With her son present we can also explore what other external resources are available to help her return to the life she wants. Perhaps they can both be helped to regain some control over their lives, and to dispel some of the helplessness.

In two or three days this can be checked out by visiting Mrs Smith at home. Many victims of violence need between one and three sessions to begin their shift from pain, chaos, disorder and impending loss. The framework not only helps the counsellor to begin to manage this, but also offers a useful model to the client.

Post-trauma syndrome

Following a psychologically traumatic event, the individual experiences symptoms of distress. This is generally outside the range of usual human experience. The trauma may be experienced alone, which is more difficult, or in groups. The symptoms involve:

- Exaggerated startle response.
- Sleep disturbance.
- Avoidance of activities that arouse recollections of the event.
- Behaving as if the event is suddenly re-enacted (particularly after an environmental stimulus).
- Diminished interest in usual activities.
- Feeling of detachment or estrangement from others.
- Guilt.
- Recurrent and intrusive recollections of the event.
- Recurrent dreams of the event.
- Numbed responses.
- Hyperalertness.
- Memory impairment.
- Poor concentration.
- Reduced involvement in life.

It must be emphasized to the client that initially these are normal responses. If they persist after 30 days they are approaching post-tramatic stress disorder. The aim of crisis counselling is to give the event some close attention in a safe environment, in order to prevent some long-term, intrusive problems.

John was brought to hospital from the police station. His friend, who had been depressed, had failed to turn up for an evening out they had arranged. John returned home but his wife had no message from his friend, and said he must have forgotten about the arrangement. Initially John agreed, but he expressed concern for the rest of the evening. His wife said he was making a fuss about nothing.

Later that evening, on getting no reply to his telephone calls, John went round to his friend's house. A neighbour, hearing John banging on the door, came out to say that he had not seen John's friend for a couple of days. John panicked, smashed a glass panel in the front door, and gained entry.

He looked round downstairs and found no sign of his friend. The house was cold, he said it had a funny smell. He climbed the staircase and at the top he found his friend hanging.

He does not know how long he stood and looked, or for how long he screamed, but he remembers running from the house. The next thing he remembers is lying face upwards on the garden path, with a policeman kneeling by him.

When I saw John he was sitting in a chair, rocking slightly backwards and forwards with his mouth on the back of his hand.

Initially he was angry at being introduced to me: 'What can you do?' 'You can't bring him back.'

He then became apologetic and tearful, telling me it was his fault and he should have gone round sooner. Still crying, he said he had loved and valued his friend, then became somewhat embarrassed and asked if I could understand that. I said how good it was that he could say that, that men often have difficulty using such words about their friends, and I valued his being able to share that with me.

John said he didn't want his wife at the hospital, explaining how she had been dismissive of his expressed fears earlier that evening.

I invited John to tell me what had happened. I would initially listen to this first story without too many interruptions or questions. It is important to listen carefully to what is said and what is avoided, particularly the more gruesome aspects. The first session usually takes at least an hour. Emphasizing the enormous difficulty of coping with this event, I offered to see him the following day.

Day 2 (session 2)

John had had very little sleep with painful, intrusive images of the incident and a funny smell in his nose. He was unable to go to work and wanted to be alone. His wife rang me to say he would not let her help him; he accused her of not wanting to hear what happened, and others of telling him he would have to forget it. He stopped trying to talk to people about what happened.

He told me the story again, with more detail. I arranged to see him again in a further four days.

Day 6 (session 3)

John described people around him becoming irritated by his preoccupation with the incident. Intrusive recollections persisted, with periods of withdrawal and an intolerance of noise. Some noises produced an exaggerated startle response. Sleep was interrupted with nightmares and waking, sweating and panicking.

I invited John to go over the incident again, and asked if he would allow me to ask some more searching questions, assuring him he could reject this more intrusive recollection at any time. He began the journey to the house where his worst fear was realized. I asked him to describe the position of the noose, and whether he could imagine how the victim felt at the time of death. John was able to do this with tears, distress and profound sadness, describing terror, fear and panic in the face of his friend. At the end of the session John felt relief at being able to express these feelings.

Day 13 (session 4)

John described his worst thoughts about the event, and had arrived at some conclusions about the condition he had seen. He said he had previously blocked these out but now he needed to share them.

His friend had prepared for the hanging by removing the loft cover and tying a rope to a beam in the loft space, probably by standing on the stair rails and banister at the top of the stairs. Remembering that the stair rail and banister were smashed, John concluded from this that when his friend stepped from the rail he did not die immediately, and kicked out wildly, smashing the wooden struts and rail.

For John this was his friend's last moment of terror, and he tried to imagine what was going through his mind during the last throes of his life. This final horror of the event was the most intrusive and painful image – a picture of the man wildly kicking out and gasping for breath often appeared out of the blue. John felt unable to share this with anyone; he desperately needed to make the picture go away.

His constant words were 'No one could begin to imagine how horrific it was, and I cannot tell them'. He described becoming more withdrawn from those around him, and the rest of the world being unreal.

Day 20 (session 5)

Most of the session was spent talking about John being let down by his wife and others, who failed to understand that he could not disengage from what he had seen. The nightmares persisted but became more bizarre, for example seeing a river turn to blood, with people he knew struggling in it.

He was philosophical about his friend's decision to end his life, and appeared to have no problems with that. The question of why it had to be John who found him, and what did that mean, took up a lot of his time. He went on to say he would not have wanted anyone else to find him.

Day 29 (session 6)

The images were still intrusive and John asked if we could go over that day again. The incident was put into the context of John's whole day. The ordinariness of the day, ordinary routine events and then the awful intrusive impact of the suicide into the day. He was becoming weary of its continued intrusion.

I was able to establish that the house where the suicide took place was now empty and was up for sale. I mentioned the possibility of our visiting it together; John was fearful about this, visibly shaking and perspiring, but agreed to think about it.

Day 31

John phoned me and said he would like to meet me at the house.

Day 35 (session 7)

We met at the house after collecting the key from the estate agent. John unlocked the door and entered the empty house. We walked round the cold, empty, downstairs rooms. John commented that his friend had gone, he was no longer there. I invited him to approach me up the stairs as he had done that night. He did so slowly, commenting that he had run upstairs on the night he broke in. John walked slowly to the spot below the loft cover and looked up. Then he slowly backed up to the wall and slid to the floor, crying and saying how sad it all was and how helpless he had felt at the moment of finding his friend, being unable to reverse the situation.

On looking round John commented about how the rails and banister were repaired and painted. Their restoration was important to John. He went downstairs and I asked him to come back up more quickly and return to the spot where he had found his friend. He did this, and then we went into a long discussion about how well thought-out and planned the act of suicide had been.

John walked around the empty bedrooms, went back downstairs to the other empty rooms, and talked about his friend and about how other people's lives would begin within this house. He then asked if we could leave, and locked the door on it all.

Day 40 (session 8)

John arrived much brighter, having had no dreams and only one intrusive image of the house, this time empty. 'He's not there any more, is he?' His relationship with his wife was better. He had returned to the scene of horror and had been as close to it as he could now be. He had re-emerged feeling intact and had engaged with life outside again. To John, his decision to leave the house, closing the door, held important symbolism. He felt much more in control.

Day 47 (session 9)

John described himself as being back to near-normality and having no intrusive recollections. Emotionally and socially he was engaging with others. The counselling sessions were brought to an end.

The horror and the gruesome aspects of this incident were a problem. John felt that people could not listen to this, and he would not have wanted them to. He had an obsessive need to review the whole incident and to allow various different aspects to re-emerge in a safe situation. Clarification of what he saw, felt and physically and emotionally experienced was validated. His need to give it this kind of attention was accepted, and he was able to pursue his search for its meaning and to deal with the more gruesome aspects.

My experience of post-trauma counselling is that the symptoms become much more manageable within four to six weeks, in up to nine sessions. Within the first 10 days, two to three sessions should take place.

'In many cases in psychiatry the patient who
comes to us has a story that is not told and
which, as a result, no-one knows. To my mind
therapy only really begins after the investigation
of that wholly personal story. It is the patient's
secret, the rock against which he is shattered. If
I know his secret story, I have a key to the
treatment.'

(Jung)

Problems in crisis work

Advocacy

After the impact of a crisis, some clients describe a particular
difficulty. This often requires the counsellor to take on a more
assertive stance and you may be uncomfortable with this more
direct approach. An example is the feelings of a woman on
hearing of the death of her teenage son, and her attempts to
see his body and spend some time with him.

'My reality was that I needed someone close
enough to reveal myself safely to who would not
take me over and do the right thing and say the
right words, and not someone with whom I
would have to behave like they were projecting I
should behave. This kind of person is rare,
therefore what I wanted was a stranger –
someone with no expectations of me.'

(Awooner-Renner)

This theme of friends and relatives wanting to rescue clients
from their immediate difficulties after a sudden death is
described frequently (Wright, 1991). The client is in a disadvantaged position. Suddenly disempowered by the event they
have some important, immediate needs which they later regret
being unable to pursue. In this crisis the counsellor, with some
insight into these needs, will need to speak up on their behalf.
People close to them, or 'the rules of the system' may work
against them. The counsellor may become unpopular and may
meet strong resistance to suggestions. For example, a policeman or a doctor may say that they do not want a mother to see
a dead, damaged child because this will produce further distress. The relatives may often feel they will have to cope with the
consequences and will decide for them.

It is important that we give people the opportunity to discuss the value or otherwise of this encounter with the dead person. If denied it will prolong the immediate counselling and subsequently make the counsellor's task more difficult. This might mean that the full potential of the counselling sessions is not realized.

By acting as advocate, the counsellor may find himself confronted with anger, hostility and further distress. Having a realistic perception of the event, confronting death and getting a chance to say goodbye offer good conditions for beginning to manage acute grief. This is the process that offers a way for the client to be healed.

Some counsellors feel they appear to be giving advice when they suggest that an encounter with the dead person is usually important. However, we must not underestimate the chaos and disorder and helplessness experienced by the client in this situation. Initially, part of the counselling is clearly focused on the present life event and on offering a framework and direction to begin to manage the crisis.

How long to counsel

As suggested earlier, crisis counselling focuses on the present life event and becoming involved with it. In some cases however, the crisis is not resolved in this way. A previous unresolved crisis or serious emotional problem may prevent the client from dealing with the present problem. Although the immediate disarray of the event may become less intense with the crisis counselling, problems persist. For example there may be a difficult grieving process following a more traumatic, sudden death. This work is much more long term.

Should the counsellor then refer the client to a bereavement counsellor? In my experience the answer is no, and I am prepared to take on these clients for a much longer period. The value of having established a good relationship with the client is a help with the long-term work, though it can also be a problem as the major focus of my work is to be available for crisis.

Too many long-term clients may not leave enough space for crisis, so time needs to be managed carefully. It is worth bearing this in mind when attempting to organize a crisis service. There are times when every client appears to have some long-term need, and the counsellor has to resist taking on an unmanageable number of clients.

Dependency

Because the crisis counsellor is involved with the client at a most intimate, powerful moment of his life, the client may not want to let go of the counsellor. Since the event produced fears of further disastrous events, the client may need you again. The conditions which feed dependency, and are worth looking out for, are:

- Friends and family live a long way away or the client is estranged from them.
- The client has had difficulty in making friends in the past, or is suspicious of the motives of others.
- The client has little affiliation with other social groups.
- The relationship with the dead person was very dependent and did not allow outside contact.
- There is a need to use the counsellor to combat loneliness.
- The client uses the counsellor as a continued link with the deceased.

Ideally the counselling will be ended by the client because the counsellor's help is no longer needed. It will have become apparent to both client and counsellor that the focus of the work is completed. To hang on to the counsellor, the client will bring new problems to the sessions, and we need to be aware of this. Is the problem a ploy to continue contact?

The tremendous strength of some of the pain experienced in crisis can cause us to regress, producing child-like needs to be cared for and comforted, which is natural. Our counselling work is to help the individual re-emerge into adult status.

Conclusion

In our attempts to care effectively for people in crisis, we have examined a theoretical framework. This should not be a constraint but should be a means of helping us to help the client to see some order restored.

Handling pain, chaos and disorder can be overwhelming for the counsellor as well as for the client. The framework helps the counsellor to begin the process of helping the client to locate resources within himself or externally. Finding self-determination and increasing self-esteem is what it is all about.

Any change or loss can precipitate a crisis. In health care settings there is always potential for change or loss, and in many cases it actually happens. Running alongside any health problems can be other situational crises, such as divorce, redundancy or separation.

Counselling focuses on the crisis, in the hope that the outcome will be a return for the client to the level at which he functioned prior to the crisis. It is hoped that the experience may produce a higher level of functioning. The nurse is an active participant in this process, working together with the client to solve the immediate problem.

The nurse is in an ideal position to use crisis counselling. Because of the nature of her work she is able to establish a degree of intimacy which is a great asset. I hope I have stressed the uniqueness of the individual and the need to work towards an equality in the relationship.

Crisis counselling has many rewards. To witness the client's struggle with difficulties and pain, and then to watch him locate resources and insights, is a privilege. We also have a lot to learn from each client.

9

Bereavement Counselling

Alun Jones

Introduction

Over the past decade issues which are related to dying, death and bereavement have been the subject of systematic exposition as a major concern for nurses. Significant changes in nursing curricular development reflect the recognition for an appropriate orientation toward grief-related issues. Nurses are increasingly demanding counselling training to increase effectiveness of communication with persons who experience a reduction in health status in response to a significant loss or losses.

The preparation for counselling practice

> These are hard demands yet nothing less is required.
>
> (Husserl)

The development of skills and competencies necessary to become a counsellor requires a preparedness on the part of the nurse for much more than an intellectual journey. There is also an emotional, ethical and moral journey. The personhood of the counsellor is involved in counselling practice and as such includes the counsellor's values and philosophy which are not easily observable within discrete micro-interactions (McLeod, 1993).

Learning to counsel requires an understanding of often complex theoretical information, philosophical approaches and dynamic human forces which influence counselling relationships. There is a need therefore for human values to constitute a belief system which underpins counselling practice. Humanistic philosophical approaches are of particular relevance – indeed fundamental to counselling relationships. Counsellors are ultimately the advocates of people who are often in deep emotional, physical and developmental crisis. Hospitals and other health care settings are frequently cradles of distress. Counsellors working in such settings are constantly confronted with their own ultimate adversary in its many guises (Jones, 1993). There is therefore a requirement for a preparation and continued support which nurtures, sustains, and enables; so they in turn can nurture, sustain and enable others who are in need of health care. Counselling practice is frequently concerned with the existential and spiritual aspects of life. Ontological concerns such as freedom, responsibility, human growth and maturation and the quest for meaning are ambiguous matters which have the potential to arouse fear. When to hold, when to nurture, when to push and when to let go are uncertain tasks for the counsellor. There is a need to acknowledge the interdependence between seemingly conceptual dichotomies, intellect and intuitive feeling, the pursuit of self-knowledge and the need to stay with not knowing, autonomy and dependency. It is essential that the counsellor is able to address the profound and uncertain nature of the counselling experience. It is, I would argue, necessary that this understanding informs all communications within the health arena. Counselling is mechanistic and reductionist when it follows theory or technique devotedly. There is potential to ritualize counselling relationships through an adherence to procedural issues. While this process may reduce anxiety, the result can be to compound feelings of despair and confusion, and increase dependency for the client. It is the imprecise nature of counselling practice which can be harnessed as a creative force for change.

Theory, therefore, should only ever inform our understanding of human distress. It should never dictate the direction of care or the outcome. Factors such as generosity, friendliness, patience, warmth and genuine interest all contribute to the conditions for change.

Moral scholarship

The counsellor's preparation for practice should be one which facilitates the development of a mature value system. To achieve this, the counsellor must be encouraged to perceive himself as a person of worth, accepted, trusted and valued. When this occurs he can begin to trust his own feelings and experiences as a guide to enabling others to understand themselves. This process provides the experiential basis from which there can be a real understanding and valuing of the need to respect others regardless of the situation. This approach is one of empowerment and rejects the notion of what Barber (1976) describes as 'paternalistic benevolence'. This is simply a situation in which the carers make decisions on behalf of the client. The counsellor's preparation should therefore be one which embraces a belief in the self-directness of human beings. It is not, in my opinion, sufficient to be guided simply by principles of respect and autonomy. There is also a need for an appreciation of the subtle and yet complex ethical and moral issues which frequently arise in helping relationships; and to harness this understanding to an approach to communication which acknowledges the unique nature of the circumstances surrounding each person's experience of loss. King (1984) believes that if the carer develops a sense of 'moral scholarship' then assimilated values will influence all subsequent relationships. This process would enable the counsellor to grow and develop both personally and professionally and in turn contribute to the growth and development of others.

Mutuality

The process of human communication is ongoing and dynamic. Wilson and Kniesl (1987) assert that effective communication is more than the simple transfer of information from one human being to another. It is a mutually negotiated series of events which is influenced by many variables. Similarly, it has been pointed out that therapeutic communication modifies ordinary communication to facilitate human interactions which enhances mental health and well-being. This view proposes that carers should be enabled to create an atmosphere which addresses a person's problems with respect, autonomy and purpose. These tasks however provide the nurse with a major challenge: to become a skilled listener, who can effectively plan and deliver care in a manner which provides the client with a healing experience.

'A part of my landscape'

In the novel *The Bell Jar* Sylvia Plath (1963) views existential fear and despair as a blank and empty bad dream; like a dead baby in a bell jar. She struggles to avoid thoughts of death and nothingness but is forced by her inner processes to confront what is for her the ultimate concern and responsibility related to living in the world. The caring professions have similarly resisted confronting their own existential concerns aroused through caring for others. They have instead comforted themselves with more pressing concerns such as the provision of physical care, organizational tasks and the rituals of caring. Anything it seems is preferable to the ontological task in hand (see Fabricius, 1991; Menzies, 1961). The reasons for the avoidance remain uncertain. It is perhaps associated with physical and emotional exhaustion, leading to a depletion of personal resources needed to provide psychological care. Various authors propose that there is an apprehension aroused through proximity to our own eventual fate (see for example Yalom, 1980). It may, however, also be related to sorrow, the saying goodbye to people who are a part of the nurse's conscious and unconscious life, yesterday's life, today's life and life tomorrow. Like Plath the contemplation of death is a part of all our landscape; our own 'bell jar'.

Not just theory or empty techniques

> Humanity does not pass through phases as a
> train passes through stations: being alive it has a
> privilege of always moving yet never leaving
> anything behind.
> (C. S. Lewis)

Bertman (1992) suggests that there is a need to assist professionals to meet the 'near impossible demands', frequent painful losses and existential issues which confront many carers in the course of their work. She argues that to Western society the word death 'burns on the lips'. The fear of death can pervade the health arena; both clinical and educational. However, the demand for a holistic approach to health care has resulted in nurses being increasingly called upon to provide counselling to patients as a component of their role as health care practitioners. There is a need to identify methods through which the nurse can develop an understanding of grief related issues, while remaining in safety from the danger of overexposure to potentially overwhelming anxiety and feelings of helplessness. There is therefore the requirement for a safe context in which the nurse can begin to understand the complexities of the emotional reactions to grief; recognize the need for effective assessment and develop awareness of the intertextuality of biographical material aroused in counselling relationships. We bring our own attitudes, beliefs and experiences to the caring relationship.

An understanding of the concept of loss is a central concern for all who are engaged in the provision of health care. A change of health status will encompass various losses to variable degrees. For health care providers it is important that we are able to recognize the nature of loss and the many ways in which it can affect the emotional integrity of the person who is receiving health care. A major task for the carer therefore is to address the concerns of the person who experiences distress in relation to a loss or losses.

This chapter will explore the emotional reactions to a significant loss and the manner through which it may be possible to enable a healthy exploration and expression of feelings and emotions of guilt. Many of the issues will be explored within the context of grief surrounding the death of a child. Of all my experiences working as a counsellor in a medical setting, this scenario presented the greatest personal and professional challenge. The chapter as such will also consider the need for support for carers and clinical supervision as an essential and integrated component of counselling provision.

Before entering into a detailed discussion surrounding loss, it may be helpful to understand what it is we mean by the terms which are in common usage. Most of us would believe we have some general idea of the meaning of various terms such as bereavement, mourning and grief which all refer to loss. It may therefore be useful to establish an everyday or broad definition.

Bereavement

The new English dictionary (1992) provides a definition of bereavement as a state of being deprived by death, to suffer the loss of the significant person. Donnelly (1990) informs that to 'rieve' is derived from the Anglo-Saxon, that what it means is to take away by force, to seize by violence. He suggests, therefore, that bereavement is best defined as a state of being emotionally robbed. However, powerful feelings of loss which result in grief can be a response to situations other than a death, for example, the loss of a part of one's body, a change in health or life circumstances, a separation from a partner, the loss of a job or perhaps the birth of a disabled child. It is also necessary to be sensitive to the many intangible losses (or those which exist outside, or at the edge of a person's awareness) which may accompany the tangible loss or that loss which is understandable and recognizable.

Mourning

A brief review of the literature related to bereavement counselling will reveal a plethora of theoretical suppositions and models of loss. While each have merit the interchangeable use of terms related to loss can give rise to confusion. It is, therefore, helpful to differentiate what it is that we mean when using the various terms. When we speak of mourning we are usually referring to the customs and rituals which allow an open expression of grief. The process of mourning will as such be influenced and shaped by significant cultural, intellectual, sociological, spiritual and perhaps even political forces. Subsumed under these headings will be other issues such as race, social class, gender and historical factors, all of which influence and shape the course of human behaviour.

An example might be to consider the intellectual dimension of mourning. In anticipation of the death of his father, the

Welsh poet Dylan Thomas began his mourning through artistic endeavour. The poem 'Do not go gently into that good night' reflects the intensity of his feelings. A Welsh hill farmer may, in response to a similar life event, mourn through allowing a field to lie fallow, or perhaps ploughing a piece of fallow land. The feelings and emotions are the same. However, the expression of those feelings and emotions may differ due to the influence of factors which I have already outlined. This is of major importance to our understanding of the need for human beings to mourn their losses in ways which have subjective meaning to them.

Lewis (1979) provides a powerful illustration of this notion. She describes an incident in which a male child was still-born. The mother on viewing her dead son took hold of him in her arms. She kissed his lips, she kissed his umbilicus and kissed his penis. She held his body in such a manner as to pretend that he was alive, walking along the floor like the toddler she would have wished him to become. She gave her son back to the nurse and wept. An empathic (and perhaps a rather creative) interpretation of these events suggests the mother's behaviour was self-empowering. The kiss to her son's mouth was symbolic of the breath of life; the kiss to the umbilicus, a symbolic link of nurturence; the kiss to the penis, a symbolic gift of pro-creativity. Her animation of the dead child was her desire for a tangible person for which to grieve. The behaviour allowed her to express her pain, give meaning to the internal and external relationships which at once existed between herself and her dead son, and provided the foundation from which to actualize her loss and begin the process of grieving.

Grief

When we speak of grief, we are referring to a process quite separate from mourning. Grief is a complex set of physical and emotional reactions to a loss (Hodgkinson, 1982). Unlike mourning there is a universality surrounding the experience of grief. That is to say, that human beings will experience similar emotions and sensations whatever the cultural, sociological, intellectual, spiritual or political influences. It is the expression of these feelings and emotions which will be influenced by the factors previously mentioned. There are of course circumstances under which there may be an absence or amplification of emotional reactions to a loss, a discussion of which is outside the scope of this chapter (see for example Worden, 1987; Parkes, 1972).

Grief is one of life's most painful and isolating experiences. For many people the period following a significant loss is one of review, both of one's life, past, present and future, and its relationship to others. Hill (1988) points out that many people are enabled to cope with grief through the help and support of families, friends and social groups. However, changes in society can separate generations both geographically and emotionally. Parkes (1972) believes that such changes can fragment family groups which in turn decreases the amount of support available to the bereaved person.

A child's death – bereavement, the nurse and the family

> After the first death there is no other.
> (Dylan Thomas)

Coping with a terminal illness and the subsequent death in a family is a profound emotional experience and can arouse great distress and suffering in the surviving family members and professional helpers. The experience can be unbearably painful. The overwhelming feelings in the face of the dying person's life fading away can be all-consuming. Feelings of helplessness and hopelessness surround the impending death.

Viewing any person's progression through illness towards death confronts us all with ultimate powerlessness.

If the death is that of a child, the dreams the family may have had for the child's future adult potential are shattered. The death of a child before its parents seemingly turns the natural order upside down. We all share the fantasy that if we live our lives in a reasonable way we will be protected from harm. Death shows this to be illusory and is replaced with a stark awareness that anything can happen at any time to ourselves and those we love. If as counsellors we are to be of help to families in this situation it is important that we have spent some time looking at the losses in our own lives and achieved some form of integration of these experiences and some acceptance of the unpredictable nature of life. The counsellor also needs an awareness of the sorts of feelings that may occur in the family and himself and an ability to stay with and facilitate the expression of these feelings as they occur. The primary role of any helper is one of companion and is never one of expert. The only expert in a particular person's journey through grief is the person himself (Cooper, 1991).

The psychological work surrounding the recognition that a child is terminally ill and their eventual death will be a physically and emotionally exhausting task. The emotions surrounding grief are documented in various ways and there are many reported examples of feelings and emotions which can be experienced by grieving people. These can include shock, apathy, disorganization, derealization, depersonalization, euphoria, denial, sorrow, sadness, guilt, anxiety, bitterness, jealousy and anger. During this time family members may also experience a regression to what Kohlberg (1975) describes as 'pre-conventional moral reasoning'. This phenonomen is characterized by magical thinking, both inhibitive and reparative. The unconscious belief is that compliant behaviour will result in a resolution of the illness. This is understood in Gestalt psychology as 'anastrophizing' and 'catastrophizing'. Simply stated these terms relate to the expectation of a good or bad event in response to the management of personal behaviour: *'If I am good in some way then ... but if I am bad then ....'* A notable feature of this process is the attempt to strike a bargain. Kubler-Ross (1987) suggests that while this can take the form of a subtle negotiation with carers, it is frequently an attempt to establish a truce with God even though there may be no acknowledgement of a God.

It is important for helpers to realize that the various reactions to grief will not be experienced in any well-defined way. The tendency to want to view the grief process in a pattern of orderly stages can have more to do with the carer needing to defend themselves against the sense of chaos and disorganization that surrounds profound grief (much like the grieving person) than is the actual experience of the parents. It is, therefore, more useful to view grief holistically and to be aware that the manifestations will be recognized in behaviours, thoughts, feelings and emotions as well as in physical, spiritual and existential changes. The reactions will be present whether faced with terminal illness, sudden death or neonatal death. Loss can often be experienced as though part of the self has died.

Prior to an anticipated death the child's parents may experience profound emotions related to guilt and anxiety, and as a result attempt to satisfy every request the child might make. This attempt to assuage powerful feelings can bring about an imbalance in the normal homeostatic family relationships which may in turn elicit feelings of insecurity both in individual family members and the family as a unit.

If the family and carers treat a child who is facing death as much like a well child as is possible, the child will in turn feel more valued and secure. An important task of counselling is to help the parents to set realistic behavioural limits that can be consistently maintained. This is a time when a sensitive and empathic counselling approach can prove invaluable in enabling the family establish a sense of mutual support.

The establishment of a healthy structure provides both the family and carers with a facilitative and protective framework which enhances family cohesiveness. It is also important to realize that no one can live with the constant reality of death and the parents of a dying child should be gently encouraged to explore the need to put time aside to renew their own emotional resources as well as those of other family members. If the dying child has brothers and sisters they will also need careful consideration. There may be problems of resentment arising in siblings through strain in the relationship with parents, who are in distress and perhaps emotionally unavailable. Qualities that the dying child possesses may be attributed to a surviving child. The dying child may be idealized by the parents and surviving children may feel resentful of this. These factors could influence the ability of all the family to express their grief openly. The surviving sibling(s) may internalize guilt believing that they are responsible for the illness and death of their brother or sister. Additional siblings may become aware of the fragility of life and fear that they may die too. This can be presented in the form of changes in behaviour patterns such as wakefulness at night. The normal homeostasis of the family can become distorted in the struggle to maintain equilibrium in the face of these secondary stresses. A family approach by the counsellor can facilitate the expression of distressing feelings by family members and increase openness in communication within the family. This can lower levels of anxiety and stress and reduce the likelihood of conflict.

If the death is sudden or unexpected there is no opportunity for anticipatory grief work and this can place the emotional well-being of survivors at risk. An example of this is Sudden Infant Death Syndrome (cot death). In these carers a healthy grief reaction can be compounded by additional feelings of guilt and self reproach. The lack of tangible explanation for the death can cause parents to review repeatedly their care for the child in the belief that they may have done something or omitted to do something that has resulted in the child's death. Listening empathically to the parents as they review the events leading up to their child's death and a preparedness to hear the same story many times can be helpful. It is also important to remain aware of the stigma associated with the often irresponsible media conjecture surrounding the cause of Sudden Infant Death Syndrome and the effect this may have on family integration and the expression of feelings essential to grief work.

Helmrath and Stemitz (1978) illustrate a number of important facts in relation to the death of a child. They believe that for many parents the death and accompanying anguish could contribute to emotional disorders. There may be fragmentation of the normal social and family support network as a result of the death. If the child suffered from a disability the feelings of guilt can be compounded as the parents may experience moments of secret relief regarding the death. This is a difficult time for carers and it is important that the death is dealt with in a supportive and actualizing manner. A further area of difficulty is that as infants have little separate identity to people other than their immediate family their death may be unrecognized by wider society. The lack of history and identity may make it difficult for extended family members and friends to relate to the parents in any meaningful way. (An example is the recently discontinued practice of providing an unnamed grave for a stillborn child; a powerful social message of the value placed by society on the loss.) The parents may feel alienated and abandoned; the loss may, it seem, be devalued.

A family approach

'Never say 'I know just how you feel'.

(Cleave)

Health care professionals can often be uncomfortable in sharing a family's loss. The parents of a dead new-born child can feel alone, the experience negatory. Simply allowing the family time to be together, knowing that there is someone there who cares can provide the basis for an important supportive network from which the family can give meaning to the event. A systemic interactional approach which involves the caring staff as well as the family can enhance healthy communication. The parents and carers should be sensitively enabled to face the reality of the child's death. This can be achieved by supporting the family while they spend time with the dead child, to hold and cradle the child in the presence of other family members, which may include brothers and sisters. The involvement of younger family members is an important aspect of care which needs careful consideration. There should be an assessment made with all of the family which involves an exploration of the feelings of all family members. This is a time when appropriate self-disclosure can be valuable and can include the counsellor's thoughts if the family asks for these. However it is important that any decisions in this matter are made by individual family members and that the choice is respected and affirmed. In the case of a young child exposure to and confrontation with death can be a case of too much too soon. The child's death awareness may give rise to anxieties. Questions related to these anxieties, may in turn, be answered by the family or by professionals in an euphemistic or evasive manner, thus laying the ground for the possibilities of future emotional difficulties. If a young child is to be included in the viewing of their dead sibling then the parents need to feel that they have the strength to deal with the child's subsequent questions in an open honest way. The family should be allowed to move at their own emotional pace and again an empathic approach can be helpful. Empathic statements facilitate the expression of painful feelings and allow an opportunity for emotional exploration and reflection. Platitudes such as 'you can still have other children', 'or you have your other children to comfort you' should be avoided. They are an avoidance of the significance of the death.

Mahon and Schreiner (1987) draw attention to the fact that when a child dies there is a considerable amount of practical organization for the parents. At a time of profound anguish they must attempt to perhaps deal with a post-mortem examination or arrange a funeral. There is also the painful task of returning home and confronting the child's nursery or bedroom. Faced with the child's personal possessions the family members can experience a powerful sense of unreality. This can result in periods of profound sorrow, sadness and in some cases depression.

The need to say goodbye

The ending of the counselling relationship is an important and often ignored task. It allows all participants to review accomplishments, acknowledge feelings of closeness, affection and anger, further loss and abandonment. During this period there is also the opportunity to close the relationship, to say goodbye and deal with the painful issue of a further separation.

A child's death has emotional significance not only for the parents and family members but also for the formal carers. Burnard (1987) supports this view and believes that helpers need to consider exploring their own emotions as part of their professional development. He believes that helpers frequently suppress emotions aroused in themselves and points to the need for opportunities for setting up support structures.

This is an aspect of caring relationships which is not yet fully acknowledged by the caring professions. It is of the utmost importance that all carers are allowed to acknowledge their personal grief in response to the death. The counsellor could provide emotional support groups and counselling groups to facilitate the healthy expression of grief (Jones, 1991). Through supportive methods of addressing their own feelings, Burnard argues, helpers will be better equipped to deal with the powerful emotions that are aroused in their clients as they occur. Worden (1987) asserts that there is a great risk of the grief experienced by all who are touched by the death of a child being dealt with by suppressive mechanisms. There may be an attempt by parents to avoid grief, perhaps by conceiving another child, or the stress surrounding the death could bring about a dissolution of relationships. For the helpers, powerful and unacceptable emotions may become displaced into personal lives or the attempt to deny grief can result in deterioration of their own mental and physical health. If, however, we can face grief then we can learn from it, to grow as human beings, a difficult and painful task for all who are touched by the poignancy of death. Parkes (1972) warns that we may choose to deal with our fears by turning away from their source, for example by jollying along the cancer patient, but he adds each time that we do this we 'only add to the fears, perpetuate the problem and ultimately miss the opportunity to prepare ourselves for the changes which are inevitable in a changing world'.

The need for clinical supervision and support

> Life is still a grand adventure, a fine show. The
> trick is to look at it and play in it at the same
> time.
> (Royal Bank of Canada)

In preparing to facilitate a healthy grief response in others, the counsellor will become aware of his own losses, both previous and anticipated. The preparation for becoming a counsellor will effectively provide a mirror reflecting the counsellor's own mortality. For this reason the counsellor should be encouraged to consider himself not only as a participant of the helping process but also as an evaluator. It is important that evaluation refers not only to the content and delivery of the counselling session but also to all of the participants' feelings. Learning to counsel requires the provision of a safe environment in which to explore, understand and express the feelings aroused through caring for others.

Formal evaluation of any counselling relationship should be organized in a manner which provides the counsellor with an opportunity to commit thoughts and feelings to a discursive level as well as to facilitate private reflection, comment and a healthy closure. This process in itself is a consciously constructed learning experience which can make a major contribution to the counsellor's own good mental health, scholarship and moral development. It is also likely to decrease the sense of emotional isolation arising from the need for confidentiality.

The provision of clinical supervision in nursing practice remains a contentious issue. Faugier (1992), for example, suggests that supervision is a concept which exists outside of traditional hierarchical roles of nursing. She believes that for many nurses, it is associated with ideas of criticism or discipline. In many instances, however, nurses and counsellors may deny their own need for support. This can be due to a compulsion toward caring, through which the carer defends against being in need themselves. The author D. H. Lawrence described this process as the 'greed of giving'. The notion of nurses being able to give constantly to others while themselves remaining emotionally and physically healthy is one of the great myths of our profession.

The idea of carers being people in need is not new. Goldberg (1986) for example believes that the choice of a caring profession as an occupation can often be guilt based and this can affect the practitioner's own recognition of the need for help. In my experience as a counsellor, carers who find themselves in distress or face personal crisis often experience considerable difficulty in accepting support. If, however, the carer is unable to accept help himself, then I would question whether he really can give help to others.

Hawkins and Shohet (1989) identify supervision as a central form of support. It is, they suggest, one in which the counsellor is enabled to focus on his own difficulties and share the responsibility for working with people who are in distress. These authors also believe that through clinical supervision, the counsellor can continue learning and development, manage workload, use personal resources for effectiveness, and learn to challenge inappropriate patterns of coping in the care setting. It is my belief that the therapeutic trajectory is often inverse. Caring for others should begin from a point within the self. An understanding of ourselves, indeed a good relationship with ourselves, is the starting point from which to develop good relationships with others. It is of paramount importance therefore that clinical supervision plays a prominent role in any educational programme which prepares nurses for a counselling role. The commonality in the practice of counselling and the teaching of it has been emphasized. Both involve interpersonal experiences which result in an increased self-knowledge and new feelings of security. The supervision relationship is a review of and rehearsal for events which occur in the health care setting.

Barriers to clinical supervision

Hawkins and Shohet (1989) suggest that in order to arrange effective clinical supervision, it is helpful to recognize the barriers which impede it, and to find effective ways of overcoming them. They identify problems such as personal inhibition, perhaps arising from practical or organizational difficulties. The latter example may not always be open recognized. The organizational message may be explicitly one of support but implicitly one of deviance on the part of the counsellor for needing that support. This can in effect reduce the overall cost of the provision and delivery of care at the expense of both the practitioner and client's emotional well-being. Hingley and Harvis (1986) support this view. They believe that although the demands of caring for others can be extremely stressful, the nursing profession often views stress as a problem for the individual and as such the alleviation of it as a personal responsibility. Bailey (1984) contends that the carers most at risk of emotional difficulties and illness are those who are particularly conscientious and committed to their work. Both authors make a strong case for a supportive forum as an integral component of health care delivery.

Rowan (1987) believes that in choosing to become carers we expose ourselves to relationships which are 'different from the normal, often engaging in a battle against the odds, leaving us drained with nothing else to give'. At such times, he suggests, it would be easy to keep one's head down, to get on with things and not have opportunity to reflect on our practice. The outcome of this could be to enter into a subtle collusion with the organization, to deny any difficulties in order to avoid the exposure of feelings of inadequacy. At such times clinical supervision has tremendous growth potential, to provide the counsellor with an opportunity to reflect on difficult issues.

As both nurse and counsellor, my own experience of clinical supervision has taught me the importance of sharing the responsibility for caring; to become aware of aspects of oneself which would normally exist outside of one's own awareness but which exert an influence on the caring relationship. My experience of supervising others who are counsellors has taught me that learning in helping relationships can never be considered at any point to be at a state of completion. It is a dynamic process and as such there is a need to create a safe context through which to challenge ourselves. This process can be harnessed as a powerful experiential teaching method. The supervisor can guide the counsellor to links and themes which (over subsequent sessions) can provide important and occasionally powerful insights into personal blind spots and defences. This would contribute to the emotional well-being of all participants in caring relationships.

A return to our landscape

> To the person in the bell jar, blank and
> stopped as a dead baby, the world itself
> is the bad dream ...
>
> (Sylvia Plath)

Aurelia Plath believed that the greatest of all gifts she could bequeath her daughter was a desire to attain perfection in all tasks which she would undertake during her life's journey. This gift, however, was to prove a burden too great for Sylvia to carry. It imposed on her an ideal which could never be realized and, as such she spent much of her life tyrannized and oppressed by internalized oughts and shoulds – psychological barriers and walls which she experienced as real constraints but which could not be seen and therefore not easily understood by her contemporaries.

It is at this point that this discussion has travelled its full circle. In the most fundamental sense, nurses who counsel in health care settings may be in danger of entrapment in a 'bell jar'. Caring for a person who has experienced a bereavement arouses feelings of distress and dissatisfaction. The counsellor is unable to give back to their person that which is really desired – the lost object. The person receiving care in return cannot give to the counsellor/carer the satisfaction of being helped (Parkes, 1972). The paradox the counsellor finds himself in can result in a powerful sense of isolation. There are also further contradictions in terms of organizational demands for throughput, the medicalized expectation of cure, the arousal of role envy in colleagues and the counsellor's own need for affirmation. This takes place in an environment in which there are frequent failures in empathy toward this demanding and emotionally exhausting work.

Schon (1989) offers by way of analogy, professional practice as a high, hard ground overlooking a swamp. 'On the high ground, manageable problems lend themselves to solution through the application of research-based theory and technique. In the swampy lowland, messy confusing problems defy technical solution.' Schon contends that it is to the swamp we must look 'for issues of greatest human concern'. Problems associated with counselling practice do not present themselves as well-defined. The attempt of precision in the delivery of health care, within an arena which is anything but precise, creates its own tension, its own conflicts. Support and clinical supervision should be planned and delivered in a way which conveys respect for the counsellor's individuality. This in turn would allow the counselling process to be structured in a manner which observes the fundamental conditions of good human relationships, warmth, genuine human respect and importantly, empathic understanding (Rogers, 1961).

The supervision process must enter the phenomenological world of the 'swamp dwellers' – counsellors and clients. It is important to avoid the assumption that the counselling relationship will be received in the same manner by each participant; to encourage and promote a capacity for reflection; to understand that some change will occur in an indefinite period; and ultimately to enhance the ability to respond to the demands which are made on the counsellor through prolonged contact with people in distress.

Conclusion

A person who is grieving sometimes needs the care and attention of a caring practitioner; nurses engaged in counselling practice need the nurturing of a caring and supportive milieu, to help to prepare for the awesome event of being with others who are in profound emotional and physical crisis. Bertman (1992) reminds us that confrontation with death not only 'evokes horror, exhaustion and separation it can also be an opportunity for existential communion'. It can remind us of the wonder of life and the specialness and connectedness we share with one another. 'Death is the backdrop against which we play out mortality and enact our humanity.' The appropriate utilization of the counselling relationship can provide a safe means through which those who have experienced a significant loss are introduced to a skilled and compassionate listener. For many people this could be the beginning of an enabling and healing experience. For the many nurses who counsel, this could provide a first step on the journey toward what Lerner (1978) has described as a 'blessed experience'.

10

Counselling Across Cultures

Peter Akinwunmi

The aim of this chapter is to address some of the factors involved when counselling individuals from a different culture. Nurses and counsellors will recognize this is far more likely in today's world than ever before. The total number of immigrants from the new Commonwealth and Pakistan is over 2.2 million, just over 4 per cent of the UK population. About 40 per cent of these were born in this country. In some of our larger cities such as London, Birmingham, Leicester, Wolverhampton and Bradford, ethnic minorities may form up to 20 per cent of the population (Brown, 1983). In addition about 1.4 per cent are from Ireland and there are substantial numbers from Poland, the Ukraine and Hungary.

Only in the fairly recent past have we come to recognize the unacceptability of failing to provide a culturally responsive health care service which takes account of very real differences in beliefs, values and norms. Consequently multicultural awareness is a growing aspect of health care.

In the broad field of nursing and midwifery, it is suggested that difficulties in communication with clients and a lack of culturally specific knowledge interferes with the ability to develop therapeutic relationships (Murphy and Macleod Clark, 1993). This is important for all nurses but particularly so for those involved in counselling. In the preface to their book, Patricia d'Ardenne and Aruna Mahtani (1989) say,

> ... institutionalised racism has meant that cultural
> issues are rarely given importance, and are often
> minimised in the counselling relationship.

To ask the question, 'What is required to develop cultural competence in counselling?' implies that counselling across ethnic and cultural boundaries requires abilities over and above the possession of core skills. This is my belief and has inspired this chapter.

It is the *attitudinal* component which must underpin any claim of competence. Moreover, the requirement for appropriate attitudes goes somewhat further than an acceptance of one's own potential for pre-judgement on the basis of ethnicity and/or skin colour. It includes an awareness and willingness to question one's own 'cultural baggage'. This is not to say that the counsellor must always compromise or change his views, rather that he must accept that culturally derived thoughts and behaviours should not be valued one against another.

Culturally specific *knowledge* refers to an awareness of the significance of different aspects of the client's culture. The main aspects are: beliefs about the self, family life and relationships; beliefs about 'helpers'; life expectations; and attitudes toward ill health and psychological problems.

Cultural competence demands a *skills* repertoire which in essence is the ability to respond congruently and appropriately to the range of minority culture speech patterns and idioms, non-verbal behaviours and all those facets of knowledge referred to above. In practical terms the lowest level of competence would mean at least having the ability to avoid causing offence. This chapter can do little more than point out some of the pitfalls; fuller texts such as D. W. Sue (1981) provide information relating to particular cultural groups and the various differences in expression. Each of these areas of cultural competence is now examined in turn.

Attitudes and cultural competence

> ... cultural knowledge of any kind is of little
> value if counsellors whether black or white,
> cannot critically examine their own attitudes
> and expectations.

This quote from d'Ardenne and Mahtani (1989) underlines the fundamental importance of appropriate attitudes. Despite the attention paid to the concept of self-awareness in the education and training of nurses and counsellors, the eradication of personal and institutional racism remains elusive (Hick,

1988; Carlisle, 1990; Sheldon and Parker, 1993). Racism in its most obvious and grotesque expressions surfaces comparatively rarely in professional arenas these days. Unfortunately however this does not mean prejudice and discrimination do not exist. The British, it is said, have always disliked foreigners.

> ... in no country in the world is the word
> foreigner so offensively pronounced
> (Zubkzucki cited in Rack)

Continued groups of immigrants to this country experience public abuse sooner or later, even those who arrive in a flood of justifiable sympathy. Rack (1982) discusses three reasons for this behaviour namely, superiority, exclusiveness and authoritarianism. To look at each of these may help us identify 'cultural baggage' and assist the counsellor to recognize areas of self deficit.

Superiority is evident in the difficulty one has trying to convince British people that things done differently abroad are sometimes better. This is as true today as it ever has been despite the media and tourism explosions which have made images of life across the world available to all. It is evident throughout British society in very diverse forms; British politicians state that theirs is the 'mother of all parliaments' and is the best example of democracy in the world. Football commentators argue tenaciously that the British Premier League is the hardest in the world. And within nursing, it has become acceptable and almost expected to scoff at ideas, theories and practices emanating from the USA. Looking objectively however, we are forced to come to different conclusions. The successes of democracies based on other voting systems are widespread throughout the world; British football's successes in international competition remain sporadic; and nursing and nurses in the USA are the most autonomous, well-respected and rewarded in the developed world. British people, argues Rack, have a ludicrously arrogant attitude based on their colonialist history. Heavy baggage indeed!

Counsellors must be aware of this heritage and its tendency to create and support attitudes of superiority based on belief in the rightness of British ways which serves to devalue minority cultures. The culturally aware counsellor must continually appraise his/her attitude to other people and ways of working with them. This means being prepared to work with goals which the client accepts but which the counsellor feels are inappropriate or at least unfamiliar. It means being prepared to use processes which cut across theoretical dogma but which are effective for the pursuit of therapeutic outcomes.

Exclusiveness involves the setting up of cliques which exclude immigrants. This is typically British and is quite different to the way America dealt with its immigration. There, the adoption of a 'melting pot' policy meant whoever came into the country was expected to prove him or herself a 'good American'. Here, immigrants were welcomed from a utilitarian perspective to do a job, usually low paid, low status and menial and/or dirty. It is as if the British were saying, 'if the immigrant must live here, he should not intrude into the heart of our society'. He can be prohibited, by creating rules and regulations, often unwritten, which support exclusive clubs and fraternities, restricting promotion within and in some cases entrance to professions, and developing neighbourhoods where the only black face to be seen would be driving a bus. True, the expression of some of these grisly occurrences are outdated, but some equally hideous modern expressions of racism are still practised, perhaps with a touch more subtlety (Stubbs, 1993).

The counsellor's awareness should start at the level of , 'how many, immigrant-excluding cliques, do I support, even tacitly by my membership or patronage?' It may be a society or association, golf or rugby club which, though it may not have a deliberate policy of exclusion, nevertheless exercises one due to its insular, unimaginative attitude and unwritten code. The reflective counsellor will look at and analyse the patterns of social intercourse he/she has with members of ethnic and cultural minorities. It is no longer sufficient defence to say, 'but they want to keep themselves to themselves'. This is little more than arrogant stereotyping and, frankly, wrong.

Authoritarianism, according to Adorno *et al.* (1950) is associated with a number of personality traits which also relate to racist views. Whilst Adorno and his colleagues did not suggest the 'British character' or any other was inherently authoritarian, the point is that the 'authoritarian personality' was more likely to be attracted to certain professions. As it happens, those certain professions are also ones which interface with the (immigrant) population on a regular basis, in particular the police, customs enforcers and the judiciary. Thus the experience of the immigrant in this and other countries is distorted by their reception and treatment by these high profile professions.

Many immigrants from the 'third world' invest considerable authority in those whose role mirrors the 'helper', 'healer' or 'wise man' (person) from their own culture. Counselling is perceived as one of these roles and considerable awareness, sensitivity and care must be taken to avoid the portrayal of self-righteousness and a patronizing attitude.

Thus far I have discussed some of the factors in British society which underpin racially prejudiced attitudes and which counsellors must be continually aware of if they desire cultural competence. Smith (1985) describes another attitudinal flaw observed in some counsellors which she describes as the 'myth of sameness'. Alexander Thomas and Samuel Sillen (1972) in their blistering attack entitled *Racism and Psychiatry* called it 'Color Blindness'. (Despite the age of this text, its principles are far from outdated). It is no virtue, they say,

> ... if it means denial of differences in the experience, culture and psychology of black Americans and other Americans. These differences are not genetic, nor do they represent a hierarchy of 'superior' and 'inferior' qualities. But to ignore the formative influence of substantial differences in history and social existence is a monumental error.

Many black people have been blessed (*sic*) with the white person's banal 'compliment', 'I treat you all the same, after all you're the same as us really'. Such statements are derogatory and insulting toward minority culture members. One would not expect counsellors to use such a phrase, at least not since the 1960s. However the attitude which lies beneath it may still carry some currency and lead inadvertently to completely inappropriate approaches to transcultural counselling relationships. The psychological needs of the black person of whatever origin, include regard for what he or she is.

Smith (1985) goes on to say that whilst empathy is an absolute pre-requisite for effective counselling it is not enough when working with the culturally different. To claim to be non-judgemental towards a person no matter what their colour, class or creed is to ignore the inevitable bias built up from years of exposure to one's own culture. It happens to all people in all countries of the world. Far better to closely examine oneself as a counsellor and as a person and develop a self-knowledge and acceptance of one's own racial conflicts and prejudices and the part your culture has played, historically and now, in the oppression of minority groups. Only then is there the chance that a genuine and healthy respect and a positive regard for ethnic and cultural differences can arise.

The knowledge base of the culturally competent counsellor

It would be impossible to expect counsellors, nurses or any health care worker to have a working knowledge of the differences in attitudes, values, language, religion, diet, behaviour and social and domestic traditions of every major immigrant group. There are however 'aspects of knowledge' which in conjunction with appropriate attitudes will prepare the worker to be effective and competent when faced with clients from a different culture. Of course there are a million and one individual 'aspects of knowledge' which can influence the counselling relationship. It is important to remember that the degree of importance of any one of them is best determined by the client. For the counsellor to assume any one aspect is more critical than another is a reflection of the attitudinal deficits discussed earlier.

We will only consider here attitudes toward the self and linguistic differences as these are fundamental to the counselling process. The breadth of material that it is possible to cover under this heading was alluded to in the introduction.

The wealth of literature describing cultural variations in the view of the 'self' clearly points to the existence of significant differences to the Western view of 'selfhood'. Studies of Japanese (DeVos, 1973), Balinese (Connors, 1982) and Filipinos (Marsella and Quijano, 1974) all discuss the existence of an 'unindividuated self' – in other words, a view of the self which is inclusive of significant others. This leads to a comparative lack of emphasis on individual autonomy and independence. In the Western view, 'personal growth', which is a desirable, almost necessary process, is likely to be pursued at the expense of familial ties. 'Unindividuation' leads to a person who does not aspire to independence, emotional detachment or self-sufficiency in the same ways or with the same intensity as people from a Western culture.

The difference this leads to may be evident in the expression of unhappiness and depression which has been the subject of much transcultural research (Marsella, 1981; Kleinman, 1977). Non-Western people, it is reported, manifest depression in bodily terms rather than psychological (Marsella, 1985). This is related to the different view of the self held, for example, by Japanese. Where Britons may use words such as 'sadness', 'despair' and 'dejection' which reflect internal states of feeling, the Japanese use words such as 'storm', 'clouds', and 'mountains'. The description of their feelings is impersonally linked to external objects. This serves the purpose of not drawing attention to the individual as a unique and distinct being. Therefore he remains part of a larger group or 'unindividuated'.

It is not possible in this chapter to relate specific details of culturally different self concepts, though an example may illustrate the point. In the Western world considerable psychological discomfort is generated by guilt. Guilt differs from 'shame' in that the former is 'felt' regardless of who knows the reasons for it. Shame is more a feeling generated from public exposure. The differences observed between cultures defined as 'unindividuated' and Western cultures which are strongly individualistic can be related to the degree of guilt or shame accompanying depressive mood states (Marsella, 1985). Where guilt is a feature of depression in Britain, it should not be regarded as a reliable indicator of depression everywhere. Neither should the comparative absence of guilt be considered as morally unsound just because the shame of other people knowing is more central to the depression. To do so is to miss the point. The fact is that within such a culture people are brought up to be less inner-directed (the Hindu Indian as reported by Rao (1973) cited in Rack (1982)). Also, within that culture the whole family will be affected by one member who for whatever reason is 'shamed' (by attempting suicide). A counselling strategy which took cognisance of these factors would be much more oriented toward 'saving face' than coping with guilt and regardless of the Western view of such a philosophy, the culturally competent counsellor would not make judgements based on his or her own culturally derived values. He or she would simply work with the significant variables, using perhaps the strength of familial ties to generate psychological support and orientate the client toward self-sustaining behaviours based on contributions to the family and the community.

The concept of self and its relation to the way we think is intricately bound up with language and linguistic differences. In many respects language moulds our thoughts and determines for us the kind of concepts about which it is possible to think. English is particularly rich in its variety of words which describe feelings, while Eskimos have supposedly more than 50 ways of describing different types of snow, and the Yoruba of Nigeria have specific words and a 'naming system' for different types of familial and other relationships. These differences should point us to the fact that every culture develops a linguistic aspect which mirrors what it considers as important and significant to its functioning. It is also the case that languages differ in expressiveness, rhythm and the way they relay the experience of reality. This latter point can be explored more fully.

Many non-Western languages are considered 'metaphorically concrete' rather than abstract (Marsella, 1985). The significance of this lies in the use of metaphors in the language, one effect of which is to use a more highly imaginal mode of representing experience as opposed to lexical or word-based models. In this respect, a metaphorical language provides a rich and immediate sensory experience of the world which is not diluted by being filtered through words which distance the understanding from the experience. The use of concrete metaphors links sensory experience and thought closely together. We therefore have three major areas of difference, each one subtle in itself but with very real implications for potential misunderstanding. The differences are: (a) the sense of 'selfhood' – one unindividuated or more diffuse, the other more discrete and individualistic; (b) internal representational styles of thought patterns – one highly imaginal the other lexically or word-based; (c) linguistic style – one metaphorically concrete, the other metaphorically abstract.

To illustrate the difference, it may seem rather quaint to us in the West to hear someone say, 'He is an oak tree', rather than, 'He is strong'. But Marsella's analysis suggests implications of greater significance. The imagery associated with the former type of speech ignores the need for logical constraints. The experience is personalized and private. This extends to a view of causality wherein all things have personal meanings. Chance events therefore are no longer chance events, they are suffuse with personal meanings and symbolism. The sight of a particular bird, the fall of a leaf, a book falling open at a particular page are all occurrences which may be perceived and valued very differently across the cultural chasm. The types of misunderstanding that lie in wait for the unaware counsellor, whose very function is based on linguistic communication, should be obvious. Notwithstanding the extremely clumsy conclusion that a client may be experiencing psychotic thought patterns, there are potential misinterpretations of the client's intellectual capacity, his priorities and his goals if his highly imaginative thinking style is not understood in its cultural context.

It may be said that the development of counselling as a profession is a result of the West's emphasis on words and lexical orientations. However in many non-Western cultures helpers do not traditionally use words to ease suffering. It cannot be under-estimated how alien it is in some cultures to rely on talking as a means of helping. The Native American (Indian) culture is one such example. It is also highly imaginal and uses a metaphorically concrete language pattern. Working with Native Americans requires an understanding of the experiences of oppression, of the feeling of 'oneness' with the universe, expressed not only in the speech pattern, but also in the non-verbal aspects of their communications with people and with significant elements of nature (Richardson, 1981). Any semblance of counselling help must be tied inextricably to the way such cultures define their values, construct their reality and the way it is communicated.

Many culturally different clients are of course communicating in a second language. This brings special problems of its own, not the least being that in times of stress the ability to find the right words in the new vocabulary is even more difficult than usual. d'Ardenne and Mahtani (1989) say that competent transcultural counsellors working across language difficulties will understand the significant limitations imposed on clients who have no choice than to use their second language. They make the point that it is good practice to approach topics in a number of ways in order to help the client elaborate more clearly.

Furthermore, there are a set of principles which counsellors should adopt when working with interpreters. The counsellor cannot assume that the interpreter's grasp of either English or the language/dialect of the client is sufficiently adequate to represent fully the sublety of meanings which traverse the counselling interaction (Shackman, 1985). Checks must be made that words such as 'feeling', as in: 'How are you feeling today?' are properly conveyed to the client. In a clumsy translation the word 'feeling' would not convey to the client that the counsellor wants to explore his emotions or moods, but rather that he is interested in bodily sensations or illness. For the counsellor to have some measure of confidence in the translator they must meet before the session(s) and develop a strategy to deal with as many possible areas of uncertainty as possible. The counsellor must be aware of the translator's non-verbal behaviour as he is of the client's and check on the translator's interpretations as assiduously as he monitors the client's level of understanding. Clearly the development of such expertise can only come with practice preferably supervised by a counsellor experienced in working across cultures.

The skills base of the culturally competent counsellor

As in the previous discussion on the knowledge base, it is only possible to convey here some broad generalizations regarding skill areas rather than an exhaustive list of do's and don'ts. Indeed the integral relationship between knowledge and skill makes the distinction between them illusory. Under this heading we will look at some aspects of non-verbal communication and the development of an overall strategy in a counselling relationship.

Non-verbal behaviour and conversational conventions, sometimes referred to as para-linguistics, are fundamental to relationship formation within, as well as between, cultural boundaries. In the initial stages of a cross-cultural encounter, the way in which the counsellor behaves will contribute to the establishment of credibility in the eyes of the client equally as much as what he or she says.

Aspects of behaviour such as the maintenance of personal space differ cross-culturally in very meaningful ways. The description of areas surrounding the self, classified into inter-personal zones depending upon distance, was posited some time ago (Hall, 1966). Hall's thesis suggested four zones: 0–18 inches, intimate; 18 inches to 48 inches, personal; 4 feet to 12 feet, social; and beyond 12 feet, public. This notion must be re-interpreted in line with cultural variations. Most African and Latin cultures naturally stand and sit closer to each other. It is not unusual for West African men to hold the hand of a good friend or even a new acquaintance if he is a family member of another close friend. D. W. Sue (1981) reports that Eskimos, when discussing intimate topics will sit close but side by side rather than face to face. Most British people would feel Africans intrude into their personal space, whilst the African would be confused by a person who tried to converse on personal topics from beyond touching distance. The demonstration of skill in this context comes firstly in arranging seating and the self in a way that will encourage the client to recognize the counsellor as a credible and sincere source of help.

Should the British counsellor, early in the counselling process, address the issue of cultural difference? This question forces us to consider some of the detail of the beginnings of a transcultural counselling session. The counsellor needs to explain his or her role and his or her belief about the way in which counselling may help. This can be especially helpful when the client's cultural values do not embrace counselling as a legitimate form of help. By giving the explanation the counsellor is setting out his or her stall. The client can then make the decision whether or not to continue. There is of course no absolutely correct way to address the fact of cultural difference in a first meeting. Indeed, a reason to talk about it explicitly may not arise. However the skilled counsellor will be looking for cues from the general conversation which will help in assessing the significance of cultural difference within the relationship.

The following example will illustrate the point. The counsellor (Ian) is a white British male, the client (Indira) an Asian female. They have introduced themselves and the counsellor has explained his role and the way he works.

Ian: So, would you like to tell me something about yourself Indira?

Indira: Well … I had to come to see you because I have been very unhappy.

Ian: Can you tell me more about your unhappiness?

Indira: (Looking to the floor). It's hard to know where to start, my family seem to see it clearer than I do.

Ian: Well let's start with how *you* see it.

What cues are there for the culturally competent counsellor in this brief illustration? First of all Indira says 'I *had* to come to see you', the emphasis being on the 'had' to. This suggests Indira feels pushed. There is a possibility it is her family who are pushing. Alternatively, or also, she may be coming to counselling from a feeling of responsibility to her family, out of duty perhaps rather than felt need. Even her 'unhappiness' may be something that has been defined by the family rather than herself. This should be followed up later in the session.

In looking to the floor while answering Ian's invitation to say more about her unhappiness, Indira may not necessarily be responding to embarrassment or a depressed mood, so much as showing a culturally consistent reaction to an older male in a position of authority. This is not to say her reaction is not an indication of low self-esteem, embarrassment or depression, but the culturally competent counsellor would be aware of the possibility of the cultural overlay and be prepared to look for other signals. Indeed the whole issue of eye contact in face-to-face interaction is another significant variable in cross-cultural encounters. Again there are differences from culture to culture which make it impossible to prescribe behaviour for the counsellor but are sufficient to make us aware of the need to adapt.

Reference to the family in Indira's second response allows the counsellor the opportunity to explore its influence. In this example however Ian follows a different line and explores how Indira sees things herself. The importance of the family and the 'de-individuation' concept referred to earlier may mean that whatever Indira thinks from her own perspective, lacks value to her, when compared to the view of the family. If the counsellor regards how Indira feels is paramount, to pursue this view may be to fall into a cultural trap, i.e. the Western value begins to exert inappropriate influence on the process. Of course at this stage neither Ian nor Indira are aware of the potential dissonance this may lead to. This example illustrates how, in a general conversation without reference to cultural differences, the counsellor can pick up cues and/or make errors.

As has already been said there is no 'correct' way to address the fact of cultural or ethnic difference. It is clearly unhelpful however to begin by posing questions which may prove to be culturally intrusive. Enquiring about a client's cultural background may be difficult to resist but the counsellor is better advised to wait until the issue is broached by the client rather than risk resistance. When necessary however the counsellor may well want to say that to understand fully the client's experience or point of view he or she needs to know more about how the way of life is for the client. What the counsellor would not do in these circumstances is to attempt to convince the client that he or she can empathize when true empathy is unlikely due to the disparity in their respective life experiences. Empathy towards a client *in the counselling situation* there and then, is different to empathizing with the life experiences of the client *as it has been lived.* Attempted demonstration of the latter is inappropriate, not to say almost impossible in a cross-cultural context.

To complete this section on skills I will briefly examine the overall strategy of the culturally competent counsellor. I have referred earlier to the need to ensure that goals and processes are consistent with the culture of the client. This comes from the work of D. W. Sue (1981) who has developed a conceptual model around these very issues.

The matrix (Figure 10.1) describes four conditions of the transcultural counselling encounter based on the appropriateness or otherwise of processes and outcomes (goals). This model provides a structure for checking if the overall strategy is culturally sensitive.

Condition 1 is the ideal scenario, where the goals and the processes are in accordance with the cultural background of the client. To illustrate this model we may consider the case of a young West African male (David) who is referred to counselling after being seen in the Accident and Emergency department of the local hospital. It transpires he has been

	G O	A L S
	Appropriate	Inappropriate
Appropriate **PROCESSES**	Condition 1	Condition 2
Inappropriate	Condition 3	Condition 4

Figure 10.1

significantly underachieving at school and getting into fights which necessitated his treatment.

A counsellor who knows that scholastic achievement is of prime importance to most West African families will realize that the expectations of the client (and his family) will be measured in large part by how quickly and assiduously David returns to his studies. The counsellor may well demonstrate his flexibility and willingness to adopt appropriate processes by working in an 'educational' mode with David, encouraging study skills for example rather than focusing on the source of his anger. When working across cultures, counsellors often need to demonstrate a willingness to move outside of the sometimes narrow constraints of the traditional counselling ethos and methodology (Calia, 1968). Thus Condition 1 is satisfied by working in an educational way toward goals that are culturally acceptable.

Condition 2 applies when a counsellor attempts to work toward inappropriate goals though using perfectly reasonable methods. This may be exemplified by the counsellor attempting to reduce David's fighting behaviour (even though such a goal may be 'agreed' between David and the counsellor). The counsellor may negotiate a series of behaviourally oriented stages which because of their clarity, their objective logic and clear relevance to part of the problem, seems a perfectly justifiable plan – a plan however which because of the goal is doomed to failure. To reduce fighting behaviour in a young black male who is in an environment he perceives as threatening and hostile is difficult enough. Added to that is the fact that his culture values displays of strength and the will to win and denigrates males who side-step physical confrontation.

Condition 3 applies when counsellors work toward appropriate goals but neglect the importance of working in a culturally consonant strategy. The current emphasis on non-directive, Rogerian techniques in the training and practice of counselling illustrate some of the potential problems in this area. The patience, the degree of introspection and the requirement for self-analysis would be antagonistic to many cultures, including David's. If the goal, to return David to his previously high level of scholastic achievement (culturally appropriate), is addressed using a Rogerian strategy (culturally inappropriate), the effectiveness of the relationship would be severely compromised by cultural dissonance. The West African culture is more responsive to a confrontational, directive style. It is what would be expected of a person in a helping role and anything less is likely to be regarded initially with confusion and later perhaps with disdain.

Condition 4 should now be obvious. To work with David towards reducing his fighting behaviour by adopting a Rogerian style would quickly lead to disillusionment with the counselling process and early termination of the relationship.

For this model to be useful the counsellor must be aware of many factors within the client's world. It is only through a sincere commitment to gaining culturally specific knowledge that the counsellor can raise his or her level of expertise. Counsellors who bother to go to the trouble of finding out about the culture of a minority group will be rewarded by the satisfaction and interest of seeing the world from a different perspective. Moreover they will find their own perceptions changed and honed. Whilst many of the things we discover remain difficult to accept, for example female subjugation, the value comes from seeing these things as part of a wider, viable social organization and importantly, feeling no right to stand in judgement.

Cultural competence demands that counsellors accept their previously robust moral stances will be sometimes undermined by new knowledge and there will be discomforts attached to questioning and re-questioning their values. It is not easy but there are always new insights, new challenges and higher levels of achievement to be gained.

REFERENCES

Adler, A. (1931) (1992) *What Life Could Mean to You*. Oxford, Oneworld Publications.

Adlerian Society of Great Britain for Individual Psychology (1991) Information Booklet, London.

Adorno, T., W., Frenkel-Brunswick, E., Levinson, D. J. *et al.* (1950) *The Authoritarian Personality*. New York, Harper.

Alderson, P. (1993) *Children's Consent to Surgery*. Open University Press, Milton Keynes.

Altschul, A. T. (1972) *Patient–nurse interaction: a study in acute psychiatric wards*. Churchill Livingstone, Edinburgh.

Awooner-Renner, B. (1991) I desperately needed to see my son. *British Medical Journal*, **302**, 356.

Bailey, R. D. (1984) Autogenic regulation training and sickness absence amongst student nurses in general training. *Journal of Advanced Nursing*, 481–587.

Bandura, A. (1977) Self-efficacy: towards a unifying theory of behaviour change. *Psychological Review*, **84**, 191–215.

Barber, B. (1976) Compassion in medicine toward new definitions and new institutions. *New England Journal of Medicine*, **795**, 939–40.

Beck, A. T. (1976) *Cognitive therapy and the emotional disorders*. International Universities Press, New York.

Bee, H. (1995) *The Developing Child*. (7th edn). Harper Collins College Publishers, New York.

Berne, E. (1964) *Games People Play*. Penguin, London.

Bertman, S. (1992) *Facing Death: Images, Insights and Interventions*. Hamispher Publishing, New York.

Boore, J. (1978) *A Prescription for Recovery*. Royal College of Nursing, London.

Bordin, E. S. (1976) *The Working Alliance – Basis for a general theory of psychotherapy*. Paper presented to the meeting of the American Psychological Association, Washington DC, September.

Brown, C. (1983) Ethnic Pluralism in Britain, the Demographic and Legal Background. In *Ethnic Pluralism and Public Policy* (eds. N. Glazen and K. Young). Heinemann, London.

Brown, M. and Fowler, G. (1971) *Psychodynamic Nursing: A Biosocial Orientation.* W. B. Saunders Company, Philadelphia.

Brykczynska, G. (ed.) (1989) *Ethnics in Paediatric Nursing.* Chapman and Hall, London.

Buckman, R. (1984) Breaking bad news – Why is it so difficult? *British Medical Journal,* **288**, 1597–9.

Buckman, R. (1992) *How to Break Bad News.* Papermac, London.

Burnard, P. (1987) Spiritual distress and the nursing response; theoretical considerations and counselling skills. *Journal of Advanced Nursing,* **12**, 577–82.

Burnard, P. (1992) *Counselling: A Guide to Practice in Nursing.* Butterworth-Heinemann, Oxford.

Burnard, P. (1994) *Counselling Skills for Health Professionals* (2nd edn). Chapman Hall, London.

Calia, V. F. (1968) The culturally deprived client: a reformulation of the counsellor's role. *Journal of Counselling Psychology,* **13**, 100–105.

Caplan, G. (1964) *Principles of Preventive Psychiatry.* Basic Books, New York.

Carlisle, D. (1990) Equal Opportunities 'given lip service'. *Nursing Times,* **86** (49), 7.

Cartwright, A. (1964) *Human Relations and Hospital Care.* Routledge & Kegan Paul, London.

Chambers, M. (1994) *Learning Psychiatric Nursing Skills: the Contribution of the Ward Environment.* Unpublished D.Phil thesis. University of Ulster.

Chambers, M. and Long, A. (in press) Supportive clinical supervision. *Journal of Psychiatric and Mental Health Nursing.*

Clark, L. (1988) Ideology, tradition and choice: questions nurses ask themselves. *Senior Nurse,* **8**, 11–13.

Clarke, A. (ed.) (1994) *Genetic Counselling, Practice and Principles.* Routledge, London.

Connors, L. (1982) The unbounded self and balinese therapy. In *Cultural Conception of Mental Health and Therapy* (eds. A. Marsella and G. White). Reidel Press, Boston.

Cooper, D. (1991) Long-term grief. *British Medical Journal,* **303**, 6802.

Cormack, D. (1976) *Psychiatric Nursing Observed.* Royal College of Nursing, London.

Cormack, D. (1983) *Psychiatric Nursing Described.* Churchill Livingstone, Edinburgh.

Cox, Murray. (1988) *Coding the Therapeutic Process: Emblems of Encounter.* Jessica Kingsley Publishers Ltd, London.

Cox, Murray. (1988) *Structuring the Therapeutic Process: Compromise with Chaos.* Jessica Kingsley Publishers Ltd, London.

Cox, M. (1978) *Structuring the Therapeutic Process.* Pergamon Press, London.

Crompton, M. (1992) *Children and Counselling.* Edward Arnold, London.

d'Ardenne, P. and Mahtani, A. (1989) *Transcultural Counselling in Action.* Sage, Bristol.

Davis, H. (1993) *Counselling Parents of Children with Chronic Illness or Disability.* British Psychological Society Books, Leicester.

De Shazer, S. (1985) *Keys to Solution in Brief Therapy.* Harper Row, New York, Guildford.

Department of Health. (1989) *The Children Act.* HMSO, London.

Department of Health. (1994) *Working in Partnership: A Collaborative Approach to Care.* Report of the mental health nursing review team. (Chairman: A. Butterworth). HMSO, London.

Department of Health and Social Security. (1983). *The Mental Health Act.* DHSS, London.

DeVos, G. A. (1973) *Socialisation for Achievement: Essays on the Cultural Psychology of the Japanese.* University of California Press, Berkeley.

Dinkmeyer, D. C., Dinkmeyer, D. C. and Sperry L. (1987) *Adlerian Counselling and Psychotherapy.* Merrill, Columbas, Ohio.

Donnelly, P. (1990) Bereavement course. *Psychiatry in Practice.*

Draguns, J. (ed.). *Handbook of Cross Cultural Psychology.* Allyn & Bacon, Boston.

Dreikurs, R. (1950) *Fundamentals of Adlerian Psychology.* Alfred Adler Institute, Chicago, Illinois.

Dyregrov, A. (1991) *Grief in Children: A Handbook for Adults.* Jessica Kingsley Publishers, London.

Egan, G. (1994) *The Skilled Helper: A Systematic Approach of Effective Helping.* (5th edn.) Books/Cole, Pacific Grove, CA.

Ellis, A. (1962) *Reason and Emotion in Psychotherapy.* Lyle Stuart, New York.

Ellis, A. and Grieger, J. (1977) *Handbook of Rational–Emotive Therapy.* Springer, New York.

Emery, A. E. H. and Pullen, I. (1984) *Psychological Aspects of Genetic Counselling.* Academic Press, London.

Erikson, E. H. (1950) *Childhood and Society.* W. W. Norton, New York.

Fabricius, J. (1991) Learning to work with feelings – Psychodynamic understanding of small group work. *Nurse Education*, **2**, 134–43.

Faugier, J. (1992) *The Supervisory Relationship in Clinical Supervision and Mentorship in Nursing* (eds. Butterworth and Faugier). Chapman and Hall, London.

Feltham, C. and Dryden, W. (1994) *Developing Counselling Supervision.* Sage, London.

Goldberg, C. (1986) *On Being a Psychotherapist, the Journey of the Healer.* Gardner Publications, New York.

Goldberg, C. (1992) *The Seasoned Psychotherapist.* Norton, New York.

Goldiamond, I. (1965) Self-control procedures in personal behaviour problems. *Psychological Reports*, **17**, 851–68.

Guba, E. G. (ed.) (1990) *The Paradigm Dialogue.* Sage, London.

Hagey, R. (1988) Retrospective on the culture concept. In *Issues in Cross Cultural Nursing, Recent Advances in Nursing (20).* (ed. J. Morse) Churchill Livingstone, Edinburgh.

Hall, E. T. (1966) *The Hidden Dimension.* Doubleday, New York.

Handy, J. (1991) Stress and contradiction in psychiatric nursing. *Human Relations*, **44**, 1, 39–53.

Harper, P. S. (1993) *Practical Genetic Counselling* (3rd edn). Butterworth-Heinemann, Oxford.

Hawkins, D. and Shohet, R. (1989) *Getting the Support and Supervision you need: Supervision in the Helping Profession.* Open University Press, Milton Keynes.

Hayward, J. (1975) *Information – A Prescription Against Pain.* Royal College of Nursing, London.

Helmrath, T. A. and Stemitz, E. M. (1978) Parental grieving and the failure of social support. *Journal of Family Practice*, **6**, 785–90.

Heron, J. (1975) *Six Category Intervention Analysis. Human Potential Research Project.* University of Surrey, Guildford.

Heron, J. (1991) *Helping the Client: A Creative Practical Guide.* Sage, London.

Hick, C. (1988) NHS Colour Blindness. *Health Services Journal,* May 26.

Hill, J. (1988) Bereavement care in nursing issues. In *Research into Terminal Care* (ed. Barnett J. Raiman). Wiley, London.

Hill, L. (ed.) (1994) *Caring for Dying Children and their Families.* Chapman and Hall, London.

Hingley, P. and Harvis, P. (1986) Bereavement at senior level. *Nursing Times,* **82**, No. 31, 28–9 and **82**, No. 32, 52–3.

Hodgkinson, P. E. (1982) Abnormal grief – the problem of therapy. *British Medical Journal of Psychology,* **55**, 29–34.

Holloway, E. (1994) A bridge of knowing: the scholar-practitioner of supervision. *Counselling Psychology Quarterly,* **7**, 1, 3–15.

Hough, M. (1994) *A Practical Approach to Counselling.* Pitman Publishing, London.

Houston, G. (1990) *Supervision and Counselling.* Rochester Foundation, London.

Hubble, M. A. and O'Hanlon, W. H. (1992) Theory counter-transference. *Dulwich Centre Newsletter,* **1**, 25–30.

Jerrett, M. and Evans, K. (1986) Children's pain vocabulary. *Journal of Advanced Nursing,* **11**, 403–8.

Johnson, R. (1980) *Recognising People in Crisis – Nursing Skillbook.* Intermed Communications, New York.

Jones, A. (1993) Death dreams and their meaning. *Journal of Cancer Care,* **2**, 190–93.

Jones, A. (1991) Curative factors experience by members of a support group for ward managers. *Nursing Times,* **86**, No. 40, p. 54.

Jung, C. G. (1961) *Memories, Dreams, Reflections.* Vintage, New York.

King, E. C. (1984) *Affective Education in Nursing (A Guide to Teaching and Assessment).* Aspen, Maryland.

Kirschenbaum, H. (1975) On becoming Carl Rogers. Dell, New York.

Kleinman, A. (1977) Depression, somatization and the 'new transcultural psychiatry'. *Social Science and Medicine,* **11**, 3–9.

Kohlberg, L. (1975) *The Cognitive Development to Moral Education. Phi Delta Kappan,* **56**, (10) 670–77.

Kubler-Ross, E. (1987) *Living with Death and Dying.* Souvenir Press, London.

Kubler-Ross, E. (1970) *On Death and Dying.* Tavistock, London.

Lee, A. (1994) Nursing in today's multi-cultural society: a transcultural perspective. *Journal of Advanced Nursing,* **20**, 2 307–13.

Lerner, G. (1978) *A Death of One's Own.* Random House, New York.

Lewis, E. (1979) Mourning by the family after still-birth or neonatal death. *Archives of Disease in Childhood,* **54**, No. 4, 303.

Lindemann, E. (1944) Symptomatology and management of acute grief. *American Journal of Psychiatry,* **101**.

Long, A. and Chambers, M. (1993) Mental health in action. *Senior Nurse,* **13**, 5.

Lueger, R. J. and Sheikh, K. S. (1989) The four faces of psychotherapy. In *Eastern and Western Approaches to Healing: Ancient Wisdom and Modern Knowledge.* (eds A. A. Sheikh and K. S. Sheikh) (Ch 8) Wiley, New York.

Mahon, C. K. and Schreiner, D. N. (1987) Premature death – Dilemmas of infant mortality. *Journal of Contemporary Social Work,* 1986: 332–9.

Marks, I. M. (1987) *Fears, Phobias and Rituals: Panic, Anxiety and their Disorders.* Oxford University Press, Oxford.

Marsella, A. and Quijano, W. (1974) A comparison of vividness of mental imagery across sensory modalities in Filipinos and Caucasian-Americans. *Journal of Cross Cultural Psychology,* **5**, 451–64.

Marsella, A. (1981) Depressive affect and disorder across cultures. In *Eds Handbook of Cross Cultural Psychology* (Triandis, H. and Dragun, J. eds.) Allyn and Bacon, Boston.

Marsella, A. (1985) Culture, self and mental disorder. In *Culture and Self; Asian and Western Perspectives* (eds. A. Marsella, G. DeVos and F. Hsu). Tavistock Publications, New York.

Maslow, A. H. (1987) *Motivation and Personality.* Harper and Row, New York.

Masson, J. M. (1989) *Against Therapy: Warning – Psychotherapy may be Hazardous to your Mental Health.* Collins, London.

McLeod, J. (1993) What do we know about how to assess competence? *Psychological Bulletin,* pp. 324–8.

Mearns, D. (1994) *Developing Person Centred Counselling.* Sage, London.

Mearns, D. and Thorpe, B. (1992) *Person Centred Counselling in Action* Sage, London.

Menzies, E. (1961) A study of social systems as a defence against anxiety. *Tavistock Journal of Human Relations.*

Moustakas, C. (1990) *Heuristic Research: Design, Methodology and Applications.* Sage, London.

Murphy, K. and Macleod Clark, J. (1993) Nurses' experiences' of caring for ethnic-minority clients. *Journal of Advanced Nursing,* **18**, 442–50.

Nelson-Jones, R. (1995) *The Theory and Practice of Counselling* (2nd edn). Cassell, London.

Parkes, E. M. (1972) *Bereavement: Studies of grief in Adult Life.* Tavistock, London.

Peplau, H. (1952) *Interpersonal Relations in Nursing.* G P Putmans and Sons, New York.

Peplau, H. (1962) Interpersonal techniques: the crux of psychiatric nursing. *American Journal of Nursing,* **62**, 50–4.

Peplau. H. (1986) Interpersonal constructs for nursing practice. Paper presented at the first Hildegard Peplau Seminar, Highland College of Nursing, Inverness, Scotland.

Peplau, H. (1988) The substance and scope of psychiatric nursing. Paper presented at the Third Conference of Psychiatric Nursing, Montreal, Canada.

Perls, F. (1969) *Gestalt Therapy Verbatim.* Bantam Books, Toronto.

Plath, S. (1963). *The Bell Jar.* Penguin Publications, London.

Powell, D. (1982) *Learning to Relate.* Royal College of Nursing, London.

Rack P. (1982) *Race, Culture and Mental Disorder.* Tavistock Publications, London.

Raphael, W. (1969) *Patients and their Hospitals.* King Edward's Hospital Fund for London.

Reynolds, D. (1985) *Playing Ball on Running Water.* Sheldon Press, London.

Reynolds, W. and Cormack D. (eds) (1990) *Psychiatric and mental health nursing: theory and practice.* Chapman and Hall, London.

Reynolds, W. and Cormack D. (1982) Clinical teaching: An evaluation of problem-orientated approach to psychiatric nurse education. *Journal of Advanced Nursing,* **7**, 231–7.

Richardson, E. (1981) Cultural and historical perspectives. In *Counselling American Indians in Counselling the Culturally Different; Theory and Practice* (Sue, D. W.). J. Wiley, New York.

Rogers, C. R. (1952) *Client-centred Therapy.* Houghton Mifflin, Boston.

Rogers, C. R. (1993) *On Becoming a Person.* Constable, London.

Rogers, C. (1967) *On Becoming a Person.* Redwood Press, Wiltshire.

Rowan, S. (1987) *Supervision – the reality game.* Tavistock, London.

Schon, D. (1989) *The Reflective Practitioner.* Ashgate, Guildford.

Shackman, J. (1985) *A Handbook on working with Employing and Training Interpreters.* National Extension College, Cambridge.

Sheldon, T. and Parker, H. (1992) In *The Politics of Race and Health* (ed. W. Ahmed). Bradford University Press, Bradford.

Smail, D. (1987) *Taking care: an alternative to therapy.* JM Dent, London.

Smith, E. M. (1985) Ethnic Minorities: Life Stress, Social Support and Mental Health Issues. *The Counselling Psychologist,* **13** (4), 537–79.

Street, E. (1994) *Counselling for Family Problems.* Sage, London.

Stubbs, P. (1993) Ethnically sensitive or anti-racist? Models for health research and service delivery. In *Race and Health in Contemporary Britain* (Ahmed, W. ed.) Open University Press, Milton Keynes.

Sue, D. W. (1981) *Counselling the Culturally Different: Theory and Practice.* Wiley, New York.

Taylor, J. and Muller, D. (1995) *Nursing Adolescents: Research and Psychological Perspectives.* Blackwell Science, Oxford.

Thomas, A. and Sillen, S. (1972) *Racism and Psychiatry.* Brunner Mazel, New York.

Trower, P., Casey, A. and Dryden, W. (1992) *Cognitive Behavioural Counselling in Action.* Sage, London.

Tschudin, V. (1991) *Counselling Skills for Nurses.* Balliere Tindall, London.

Tyson, G. A., Lambert, W. G. and Beattie L. (1995) *The quality of psychiatric nurses' interactions with patients: an observational study,* **32**, 1, 49–58.

United Kingdom Central Council for Nursing, Midwifery and Health Visiting. (1994) *The future of professional practice: the council's requirements for post-registration education and practice.* UKCC, London.

United Kingdom Central Council for Nursing, Midwifery and Health Visiting. (1992) *Code of Professional Conduct.* UKCC, London.

Watts, A. (1993) The meaning of happiness: the quest for freedom of the spirit. In *A Detailed Study of the Relationship between Teaching, Support, Supervision and Role Modelling for Students in Clinical Areas: Research Highlights* (eds E. White, S. Davis, S. Twinn and E. Riley). English National Board for Nursing, Midwifery and Health Visiting, London.

Williams, E. A. (1994) In *Genetic Counselling, Principles and Practice* (ed. A. Clarke). Routledge, London.

Worden, J. W. (1987) *Grief Counselling and Grief Therapy.* Tavistock Publications, London.

Yalom, I. D. (1980) *Existential Psychotherapy.* Basic Books, New York.

Wright, B. (1993) *Caring in Crisis* (2nd edn). Churchill Livingstone, Edinburgh.

Index